C. Leigh Broadhurst PhD

Prevent, Treat and Reverse
Diabetes

Nutritional guidelines
for Type II diabetics

alive
books

Vancouver
Canada

D1042890

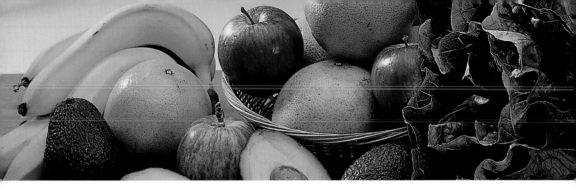

c o n t e n t s

Note: Conversions in this book (from imperial to metric) are not exact. They have been rounded to the nearest measurement for convenience. Exact measurements are given in imperial. The recipes in this book are by no means to be taken as therapeutic. They simply promote the philosophy of both the author and alive books in relation to whole foods, health and nutrition, while incorporating the practical advice given by the author in the first section of the book.

Recipes

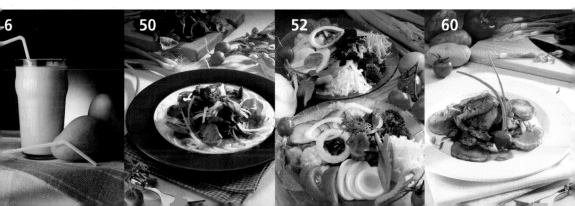

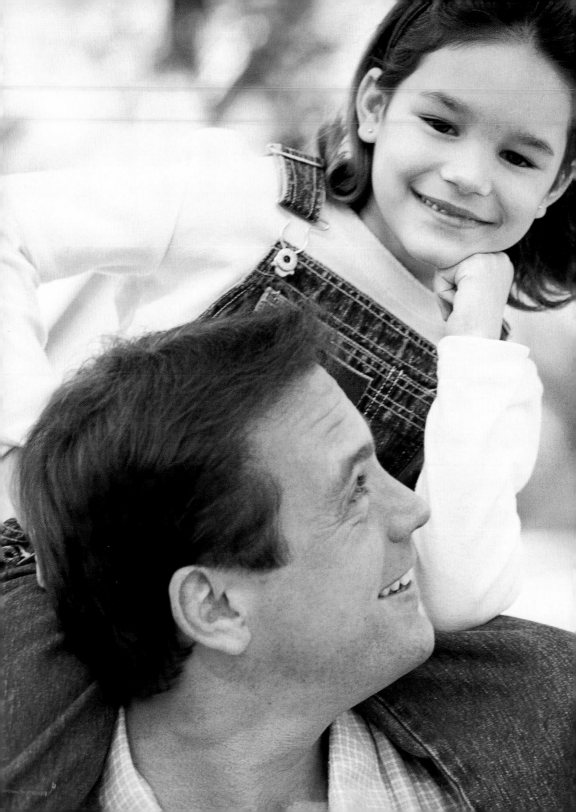

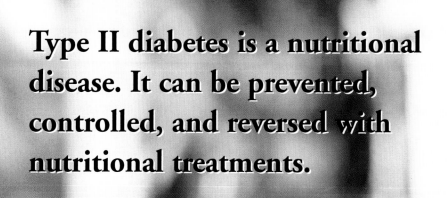

Type II diabetes is a nutritional disease. It can be prevented, controlled, and reversed with nutritional treatments.

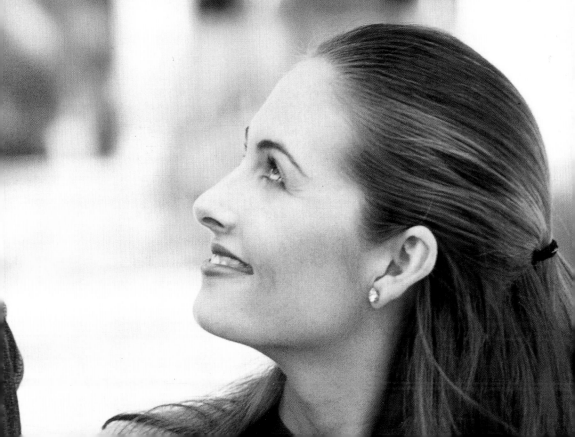

Introduction . . . .

On the topic of diabetes, there is good news and bad. The bad news is that diabetes is one of the largest health problems in North America, Australia, and Europe, and its incidence is increasing despite continual advances in medical care. Approximately 20 million Americans and Canadians now have Type II diabetes, and it's estimated that millions more are diabetic but haven't been diagnosed yet. The major cause of Type II diabetes is obesity, or, more accurately, over consumption of carbohydrates. Many new cases of diabetes are occurring not only in the elderly, but in overweight children and young adults. It is now a disease that can strike at any age.

The good news is that Type II diabetes is a nutritional disease, so it can be prevented, controlled, and even reversed with nutritional treatments. In this book you'll learn which foods, vitamins, trace elements, and herbs can be used to safely and effectively prevent and treat Type II and pregnancy-related (gestational) diabetes. You'll also learn how being lean and exercising can permanently improve your blood sugar control. If you have Type I diabetes, your condition is irreversible, but you can still look to nutrition to reduce your insulin dosages, minimize complications and greatly improve your quality of life.

The incidence of diabetes is increasing despite continual advances in medical care.

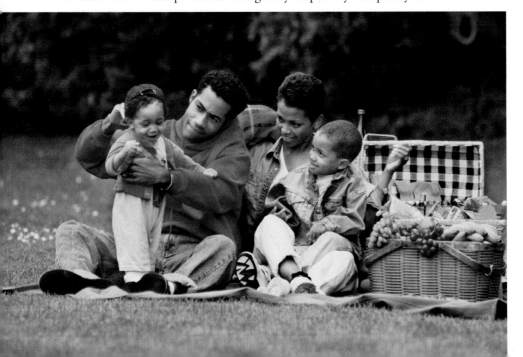

Glucose (blood sugar) is the body's primary fuel, so its regulation is crucial to our metabolisms. The hormone insulin normally takes care of this regulatory job; but if you're diabetic, insulin doesn't function correctly or else it is lacking. And if insulin doesn't do its job, one's entire body doesn't function the way it should!

If you have diabetes, your abilities to feed, grow, repair, detoxify, and heal your body are all compromised all the time. Poor blood sugar control increases your risk for diabetic complications, which include heart and kidney disease, nerve damage, and blindness.

Unlike improving nutrition and physical activity, drugs cannot reverse your diabetes. Antidiabetic medications can effectively lower glucose, but they do so at the cost of damaging your liver and reducing your life span. Some of these medications deplete your body of B vitamins and antioxidants, which brings about additional problems.

If you have diabetes, you owe it to yourself and your family to give diet, exercise, and supplements a serious try. You've nothing to lose but body fat, and you stand to gain many healthy years of life. If you don't yet have diabetes, but think you're at risk for it, you can ensure that you'll never get it by following the preventive advice in this book.

You might wonder if I wrote this book because I'm a diabetic. The answer to this is "no," and nobody in my family is a diabetic now either.

My grandfather was not at all overweight, but did develop diabetes about age 60. He died when I was a teenager, after suffering from cancer for years. It was not until a decade or so later that I began to see the link between his diabetes, cancer, and his life-long career running a hardware store. He neither smoked nor drank, yet exposed himself to pesticides, herbicides, solvents, gasoline, kerosene, and lead paint on daily basis.

Today we take better precautions to avoid exposure to environmental toxins, yet we do little to protect ourselves from the equally toxic effects of overeating, poor nutrition, and lack of exercise. The result is that the incidence of Type II diabetes is sky-rocketing with no end in sight.

The reason I wrote this book is because I've had a strong research interest in diabetes for years. I have my PhD in geo-chemistry and physical chemistry. I spend my "down and dirty" work as a scientist running analytical equipment and designing and building research laboratories. The use of chromium, medicinal plants, and polyunsaturated fats for diabetes are among the areas that I currently work in. I quickly realized that I couldn't let our research concepts and conclusions "trickle down" to the public over the course of years or even decades. We all need as much information as we can as fast as possible to prevent diabetes today. It's already far beyond the capability of any medical establishment or government health organization to control. Only YOU can make a difference.

While giving you the science in an understandable form is my top priority, there's nothing in this book that I have not tried or created myself, and tried out on others as well. I'm a speaker, writer, and consultant in the natural products industry. I've helped hundreds of people get on diets where they can finally lose body fat, and if they're interested, gain muscle. I've also helped people with Type, I, Type II, and gestational diabetes control or reverse their condition. I know what I have to say here can truly help people, provided they're ready to help themselves.

What Causes Diabetes? . . . .

Diabetes is a condition in which the concentration of glucose (a sugar) in the bloodstream is both chronically higher than normal and poorly regulated. Glucose is our body's primary fuel. All the carbohydrates we eat are eventually broken down to glucose by the processes of digestion and absorption. Carbohy-drate foods are sugars and starches–the easiest foods for the body to make glucose from. However, proteins and fats can also be used to make glucose. When you hear the term "blood sugar," it's referring to the concentration of glucose in the bloodstream.

There are several types of diabetes, which we'll discuss individually. But in all types of diabetes, a problem exists with the function and/or levels of insulin. Insulin is a hormone secreted by special cells (beta cells) in the pancreas. Insulin's primarily role is to "escort" glucose in the bloodstream, transporting it to our body's cells to provide them with energy. It also signals the cells to take in the glucose when it arrives. If the insulin system doesn't function optimally, glucose builds up in the bloodstream, yet the cells may be "starved" for energy.

Insulin also escorts proteins and fats to cells. We can't build and repair muscles, for example, without the action of insulin. This crucial hormone also helps regulate the storage and release of body fat and glycogen. Glycogen is made up of many glucose molecules linked together. Our liver and muscles store glycogen for energy, but that amount is enough to run the body for less than a day–our main source of stored energy is body fat. Glycogen is used for short bursts of intense activity, such as lifting a heavy weight or sprinting 100 meters. When glycogen is depleted by exercise or stress, insulin helps build up the supplies as soon as food is eaten. If insulin doesn't do its job, glycogen may not be stored or used correctly, resulting in extreme fatigue and muscular weakness.

What is Type I Diabetes?

Five percent of diabetics have Type I diabetes, also known as "insulin-dependent diabetes mellitus." Type I diabetes is an irreversible disease, which runs in families to some degree as it is partly inherited. It is believed that Type I diabetes is caused when a complex, abnormal reaction of the immune system attacks the pancreas. The beta cells of the pancreas become dysfunctional, producing little or no insulin. Type I diabetes typically appears early in life, in childhood or teenage years, so it is often called "juvenile onset diabetes."

Type I diabetes is also known as "insulin-dependent diabetes mellitus."

Those with Type I diabetes need to inject insulin daily to remain alive. They cannot reverse their condition, but they can certainly lower their insulin requirements, and dramatically improve their quality of life by following a nutrition and exercise program.

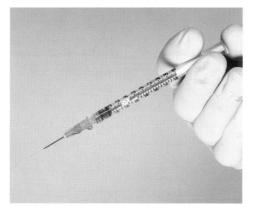

What is Type II Diabetes?

Ninety-five percent of diabetics have Type II diabetes, which is also called "non-insulin dependent diabetes mellitus." Type II is also known as "adult-onset diabetes," since it usually occurs in people over age 40.

Type II diabetes differs greatly from Type I diabetes. Type II diabetics typically have an adequate amount or too much insulin, but this insulin is not utilized effectively. Insulin receptors on many of the body's cells may not "accept" insulin correctly, or perhaps the cells have fewer receptors than they should. The end result is that both insulin and blood sugar tend to be abnormally high, especially after meals.

Type II diabetes is considered a nutritional disease because it is almost entirely caused by obesity, poor nutrition, and lack of exercise. A greater risk for developing Type II diabetes can run in families or ethnic groups, but the disease itself is not inherited. For these reasons, with a good effort on your part to follow a nutrition and exercise program, Type II diabetes can be controlled and even completely reversed.

10

Insulin Sensitivity and Glucose Tolerance

In order to understand diabetes, we need two definitions. Insulin sensitivity indicates how well tissues react to insulin. Type II diabetes is characterized by poor insulin sensitivity, meaning that tissues aren't responding to the hormone correctly or efficiently. These tissues may be described as being insulin resistant, indicating their cells don't respond to insulin's signals to take up nutrients from the bloodstream as well as they should.

If you are insulin resistant, then abnormally high levels of insulin are circulating in your bloodstream. This increases your chances of developing heart disease, high blood pressure, obesity, and chronic inflammatory conditions, as well as diabetes.

What Else Causes Diabetes?

A third type of diabetes, called "gestational diabetes mellitus," can occur in the last trimester of pregnancy. Gestational diabetes is similar to Type II diabetes in its origin and treatment, but it is temporary and usually disappears soon after childbirth. Treatments comprising dietary control and vitamin and trace element supplements are of the utmost importance in gestational

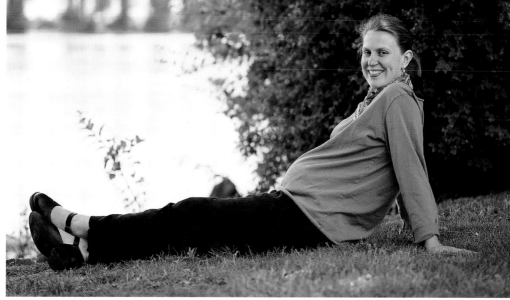

diabetes, since many drugs and herbs are not safe to use during pregnancy.

"Gestational diabetes mellitus" can occur in the last trimester of pregnancy.

Drugs such as corticosteroids can cause temporary but severe diabetes. Abnormally high levels of blood sugar can also be a symptom of liver and kidney disease, adrenal gland dysfunction, cancer or severe nutritional deficiencies. In addition, poisoning from cyanide compounds or heavy metals, and bacterial, fungal, and viral infections can damage the pancreas. Childhood obesity and rare genetic conditions can result in Type II diabetes developing between ages 10-30.

Symptoms of Diabetes . . . .

People who are developing Type I diabetes tend to experience rapid weight loss coupled with severe muscle wasting, and they have very high levels of glucose in their urine. They may experience extreme hunger, as well as tremendous mood swings–from irritable and edgy to dizzy and close to passing out. Left untreated, Type I diabetes results in coma and death.

By contrast, people who are developing Type II diabetes are likely to be overweight, but they're having no success at "dieting." They may or may not have high levels of glucose in their urine. They often feel fatigued or drowsy, especially after meals, but are not in danger of passing out. Type II diabetes can in fact produce no recognizable symptoms until it is has fully progressed.

It's very important to get a complete medical examination if you suspect you have diabetes!

Symptoms of Diabetes

- excessive thirst
- frequent urination
- blurred vision
- dry scaly skin
- fluid retention (especially in the legs and feet)
- poor healing of skin wounds
- impotence
- numbness and/or tingling in the extremities
- decreased tolerance to cold
- rapid weight gain or loss
- irregular or rapid heart rate
- extreme fatigue
- abnormal muscle weakness
- chronic itching

Diabetes Is Dangerous . . . .

We all know that a car engine can't run without any gasoline, but it also can't run with too much fuel–when the engine is "flooded." A car engine needs a precise amount of fuel, delivered at a constant rate. Our bodies work the same way, preferring to function with a steady, even level of blood sugar delivered to the cells. The normal condition for humans is a blood glucose concentration between 80 and 120 milligrams per deciliter.

People with diabetes suffer premature aging of the cardiovascular system, kidneys, eyes, and immune system. Think of how a baby's smooth, flexible skin eventually turns into the wrinkled skin of the elderly. This tissue aging is going on inside your body as well, but if you have high levels of blood sugar, it's happening much faster than it should!

Diabetes also causes premature aging by reducing immunity, while at the same time increasing blood pressure, insulin levels and oxidative stress. "Increased oxidative stress" means a greater number of destructive oxygen-free radical molecules are produced in the body, and a person's susceptibility to tissue damage from the free radicals may also be greater. Associated with this premature aging package are a number of serious health conditions, called "diabetic complications." Diabetic complications include heart and kidney disease, stroke, poor circulation, difficulty walking or exercising, deterioration of vision, and nerve damage. Complications worsen with decreasing blood sugar control and increasing age and obesity. Diabetics who are nutrient deficient, and who use tobacco or drink alcohol, have an increased risk for complications.

If you have Type I diabetes, some complications will eventually arise, but you can defer their onset and minimize their impact on your health by following the advice in this book and seeing your doctor regularly. This is especially relevant for parents of diabetic children. As a parent, you need to consider that your child is facing a lifetime of insulin injections and compromised health. In order to ensure that your child can grow to adulthood as healthily as possible, you need to start preventing complications now.

The Ideal Diet for Diabetics . . . .

Diet is crucial to control, reverse, or prevent diabetes. Volumes are written on this topic–all you need to know–but following the advice is the key! In North America we have cheap, tasty, abundant food available all the time; consequently, we are the fattest and most diabetic people in the world. "Just saying no" to excessive eating is part of the solution–but so are picking the right foods, and turning more of our bodies into muscle instead of fat. In order to prevent or treat diabetes, your number one task is to maintain normal body weight through a healthy diet and regular exercise.

Controlling, reversing, and preventing diabetes are directly related to diet.

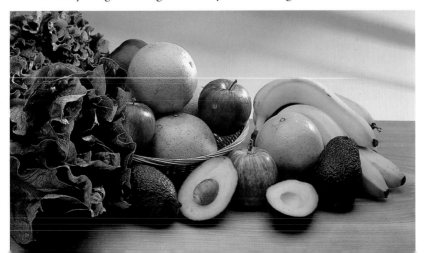

Ideal Diet for Diabetics

Here's ten simple modern diet concepts for diabetes prevention and treatment that everyone can use:

1. Eat frequent small meals. Eat five or six mini-meals each day, or three meals and two snacks. Don't starve yourself during the day, then eat a huge meal at night.

2. Each meal should be a balance of protein, carbohydrate, and fat, such as a chicken and corn on the cob. Never eat carbohydrate foods such as candy, bread, or pasta alone, and this even includes fruit.

3. As an ideal, limit carbohydrates to fruits and starchy vegetables such as peas, corn, lima beans, winter squash, potatoes, and beets. Dried cooked beans are okay, but they're a carbohydrate, not a protein food!

4. As an ideal, processed grains and refined flours should be minimized or eliminated from your diet. This includes pasta, white bread, waffles, pancakes, grits, noodles, white and puffed rice, snack chips, and crackers. Eat natural whole foods.

5. Sugar and sugary foods are big problems for diabetics of all types. The worst foods ever invented for diabetics are donuts! Avoid candy, cookies, cakes, pastries, ice cream, frozen yogurt, soda, fruit juices, etc.

6. Always consume your daily protein requirement (see "Proper Protein is Crucial" on page 17).

7. Use quality fats as opposed to refined, processed fats such as margarine and shortening. Eat a moderate amount of higher-fat fresh foods such as nuts, avocados, meats, fish, and dairy products. Use cold-pressed unrefined vegetable oils. Aim for getting about 3 to 6 percent of your total calories from polyunsaturated fatty acids from both the omega 3 and omega 6 families.

8. Choose a high-fiber diet, and use a fiber supplement, too. High fiber foods include whole grain cereals, brown rice, bran, nuts, seeds, beans, lentils, peas, and fresh raw vegetables.

9. Eat plenty of fresh vegetables. They will reduce the need for insulin and lower the level of fats in the blood.

10. Sip water all day.

Get Off the Carb-Crash Cycle . . . .

Frequent smaller meals keep blood sugar levels more even and reduce our tendency to store calories as fat. Eating protein, fat, and carbohydrate together slows and normalizes digestion and absorption, admitting glucose into the bloodstream in a steady dribble instead of a fast flow. Carbohydrates are much easier for the body to turn into glucose than are protein and fat. A big dose of sugar or refined starch (especially on an empty stomach) literally floods the bloodstream with glucose, which then causes insulin levels to skyrocket. After the "dose" is digested, blood sugar crashes and hunger and carbohydrate cravings return with a vengeance. This cycle is repeated daily by consuming candy, soda pop, pasta, rice cakes, muffins, bagels, crackers, etc. for snacks or meals.

Repeating this "carb-cycle" is unhealthy for everyone–especially diabetics–because it causes such uneven levels of blood sugar and insulin. If you are insulin-dependent, eating a balance of protein, carbohydrate and fat can make it easier to get your insulin dosages correct. An appetizer of nuts and mineral water with lemon, followed by grilled salmon, fresh peas, green salad, and raspberries with a little sugar-free frozen yogurt or heavy cream would be an example meal. If you are trying to lose body fat, if you have very high blood sugar after meals, or if you have difficulty getting your insulin dose right, you don't need to eat carbohydrates at each mini-meal. Many of your mini-meals can be all protein, or protein plus fat. Good choices for snacks or smaller meals are sports nutrition bars, blender drinks, chef's salad, trail mix, tuna or chicken salad, and fruit yogurt.

Sugar and white flour products should be strictly avoided by those with diabetes.

Carbohydrate Foods to Avoid

Most diabetics know they need to avoid sugary foods. This includes candy, cookies, cakes, sodas, pastries, honey, syrups, most fruit juices, ice cream, frozen yogurt, and other desserts. But sugar is also a major ingredient in breakfast cereals, muffins, sweetened yogurt, barbecue

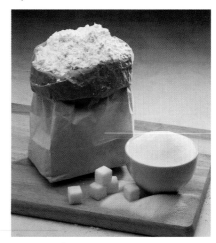

sauce, low-fat salad dressings, steak sauce, instant coffees, catsup, pickles, "beer nuts," etc. As an ideal, sugary foods should be minimized in your diet.

Worse than sugar is white wheat flour. Many people eat wheat flour two to five times per day, every day. White bread is obvious here, but rye, oatmeal, multi-grain, and corn breads are mostly made of white wheat flour as well. Most commercial "whole wheat" baked goods contain only small amounts of whole wheat. Pasta is the same as white bread–only worse, because it's eaten in larger servings! As an ideal, pasta, most breads, noodles, cream of wheat, crackers, pancakes, waffles, and pretzels should be minimized in your diet. The simplest carbohydrate rule for the diabetic diet is: "If it's sugar-sweet or made of wheat, don't eat!"

Better Carbohydrate Choices

It's far better to eat starchy vegetables than to consume starches from the foods mentioned above. Fresh fruits and vegetables are 80 to 90 percent water and are rich in fiber, which means they are diluted sources of carbohydrates. Sure, a potato has carbohydrates, but unless it's a potato chip, it's still mostly water. Not many people will eat three baked potatoes at one sitting, but three dinner rolls are no problem. Good examples of starchy vegetables to eat include corn, white and sweet potatoes, winter squash, beets, peas, jicama, yucca, and fresh beans, such as limas.

Whole fresh fruits are better choices than fruit juices or cooked fruits, but many diabetics shouldn't eat more than four servings of fruit per day. Oatmeal and oat bran are the best grains for diabetics. Unsweetened bran cereal, cooked dried beans, brown rice, cooked whole grains, and 100 percent whole grain breads are also acceptable choices.

Starchy vegetables are the best carbohydrate choices.

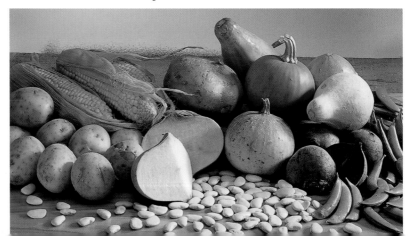

Kicking a Sugar or Starch Addiction

If you are a sugar or starch addict, and feel that there is no way you can stop eating these foods every meal, you'll need several days of intensive work to handle this addiction. First, get all the foods you cheat on out of the house! Tell yourself that if you want something terribly you can have it, but you must get in the car and go out to get it. Have healthier snacks or snacks that are not your favorites around the house instead, such as fruit, nuts, and raw vegetables.

Whenever you have cravings for sugar or starch, drink a large glass of cold water or plain tea with two tablespoons of raw apple cider vinegar or lemon juice. Also, slowly eat a little bit of plain protein, like a few hard-boiled egg whites, plain chicken, or tuna. A little bee pollen can help as well. Keep busy, to keep your mind off your craving. After 15 minutes, if the craving is still strong, do the same thing again. Repeat a third time if necessary. After 15 more minutes you'll be feeling better.

If you still have the craving and can't control it, you must get into your car and go out to buy what you crave–although it barely seems worth all this trouble. Even if you do succumb to temptation you will not "pig out" nearly as badly as usual.

Eventually, sugary treats will taste unnaturally sweet to you. For the first two to four days this will be hard, so don't even try to count calories–just follow the plan. Eat as much protein as you can handle. I guarantee that if you really avoid the "sugar siren song" in this manner you will diminish your cravings in a matter of days, and attempts at dieting may finally begin to be successful.

Please Note: If you have absolutely no success with this regimen, and tend to have "hypoglycemia" and other health problems as well, you may have a systemic Candida yeast infection and/or food allergies. Please consult references and seek professional help.

Proper Protein Nutrition Is Crucial . . . .

Everybody has a minimum daily protein requirement based on lean body mass, activity level, and state of health. For most North American adults it's between 50 and 150 grams per day. Protein is the anchor of your diet–you cannot thrive without it; you can merely survive. Unlike fat and glycogen, protein is not "stored up" one day and used the next.

If you don't eat adequate daily protein your body will cannibalize its own muscle structure, which you never want to happen. Muscle wasting is a symptom of severe or uncontrolled Type I diabetes, a situation in which insulin levels are so low that glucose can't be used for energy, so muscle is burned instead.

It's generally okay to eat more protein than your minimum requirement, so long as it's lean. If you are diabetic, you can help control your blood sugar and lose body fat just by replacing some carbohydrates with protein. Humans evolved eating a large amount of calories from protein. If we are healthy, we can eat 400 grams of protein per day before there are any negative effects. Almost nobody eats 400 grams of protein per day anyhow, except some professional athletes.

Please Note: If you have kidney disease or dysfunction, or if you are a Type I diabetic on a protein-restricted diet, please follow your doctor's recommendations regarding your protein intake.

Good Protein Choices

The following items are good choices for lean protein foods. They are listed in approximate order from highest quality to lowest quality and best to worst. All of these choices are good choices, and you can mix them up in any variety that suits you. You might also want to try some of the high protein sports nutrition bars and meal replacement drinks that are available on the market. Look for bars with at least 12 grams of protein per 200 to 300 calories of bar, and drinks with 20 grams or more protein per serving. This will provide a good ratio of protein, fat, and carbohydrate in one package.

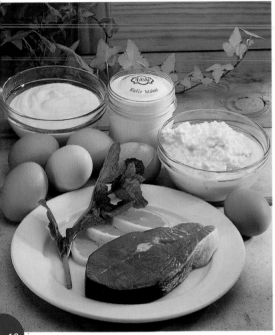

18

Good protein choices include eggs, fish, and fermented milk products such as kefir.

1. cold-processed whey protein powder
2. egg white or egg white protein powder
3. fish
4. shellfish
5. skinless organic poultry
6. game meats such as venison and buffalo
7. lean organic red meat
8. whole eggs
9. low-fat deli meats
10. low-fat cottage cheese
11. other dairy products
12. tofu and other soy products

> **Beans and Grains for Complete Protein?**
> Combining beans and grains is a semi-starvation, subsistence agriculture eating strategy, not a strategy for losing fat, gaining muscle or preventing or reversing diabetes. Beans and grains count only as carbohydrate foods, not as protein foods.

Facts on Fats . . . .

High fat diets cause or contribute to diabetes. Most diabetics are healthiest when they're eating no more than 30 percent of calories from fat. If you have too much body fat, high blood pressure, cardiovascular disease or high triglycerides, definitely aim for 20 to 30 percent of calories from fat. Diets with 10 to 15 percent of calories from fat are not beneficial, and they result in overeating carbohydrates.

Within your 20 to 30 percent fat calories, choose about one-third each of saturated, monounsaturated, and polyunsaturated fats. Diets that are high in saturated and trans-fats are the worst for diabetics, and make blood sugar and insulin regulation more difficult. You don't have to completely avoid animal fat, but don't eat it in excess.

Trans-fats are also called "hydrogenated oils." Trans-fats are artificially solidified oils that look and act like saturated fats. Trans-fats are found in margarine, shortening, fried and snack foods, commercial baked goods, and candies. Although trans-fats may be listed as "polyunsaturated" on labels, they are counted as saturated fats in your diet, and are best avoided.

The highly processed oils in supermarkets are the fat equivalents of white sugar–just empty calories. Shop at health food or specialty grocers for unrefined, cold-pressed oils like flaxseed, extra virgin olive, sesame, and walnut. Even better, consume fats in whole foods such as nuts, olives, avocados, fish, shellfish, and eggs.

If you're not overweight, yet have poor blood sugar control, you might want to consult a professional about a high monounsaturated fat diet. In this diet, calories from monounsaturated fat are exactly substituted for some of the calories in the diet that were being provided by carbohydrates and, to a lesser extent, trans and saturated fats. In practice, this means eating nuts, avocados, olives and their oils instead of carbohydrate foods. If the diet simply has monounsaturated fat added to it, there's no benefit, and you're likely to gain body fat.

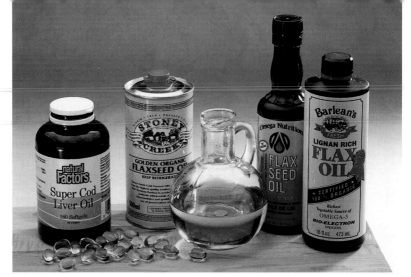

Essential fatty acids improve glucose tolerance.

Keep in mind that when you substitute fat calories for carbohydrate calories, you will be eating smaller portions of food, and you will still not be eating pastas, white breads, crackers, pastries, rice, cookies, etc. This diet is not a viable option for those with nut allergies.

Essential Fatty Acids

Essential fatty acids are essential to the body because the body does not produce them on its own—hence the term "essential." You must incorporate essential fatty acids into your diet; they are the building blocks of all cells in the body, including those in all your organs, your muscles, your skin, your eyes and your brain.

Cell membranes that are flexible have more and better insulin receptors, which improve glucose metabolism. Essential fatty acids make cell membranes more flexible, whereas saturated fats make them stiffer. This means that a diet that's high in saturated fats and/or hydrogenated fats can directly cause diabetes. It also means that adequate amounts of essential fatty acids must be included in your diet to help prevent and treat diabetes.

To potentially improve glucose tolerance, take 2 to 4 grams fish oil, and 3 to 6 teaspoons of flaxseed oil per day. Also substitute fish or shellfish for meat often, and cut back on saturated fats.

Choose a High-Fiber Diet . . . .

High-fiber diets are recommended for all diabetics. Particularly important is soluble fiber, found mainly in fruits, vegetables and some seeds. Insoluble fiber is more characteristic of brans and husks of whole grains (i.e., wheat bran, bran cereal, brown rice). Soluble fibers include pectins, gums, and mucilages, all of which slow or reduce the absorption of glucose. If you think of how pectin gels fruit juice into jelly, which is still soft, but definitely not liquid, you can imagine how soluble fiber might act in your intestines.

A high-fiber diet is also believed to help prevent Type II diabetes. Several studies have shown that diets rich in whole grains, fruits, and vegetables result in a decreased incidence of diabetes in a given age group as opposed to diets rich in white flour, white rice, other refined grains and sugars. A diet with plenty of raw or lightly cooked vegetables will provide soluble and insoluble fiber. Two studies (1998, 1999) showed that five grams psyllium seed given with each of two or three meals per day for six to eight weeks reduced blood sugar after meals by up to 19 percent.

Freshly ground flaxseed (an electric coffee grinder works well), fenugreek, and citrus and apple pectin supplements are easy ways to add extra fiber to your diet. On occasion, psyllium causes allergies or flatulence.

Obesity interferes with normal glucose metabolism and decreases insulin sensitivity.

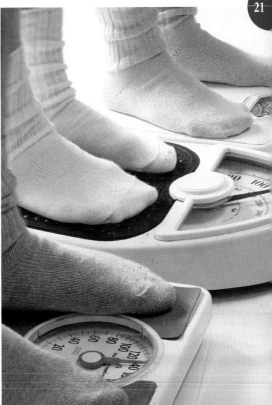

21

A Weighty Issue . . . .

Obesity is unquestionably the major cause of Type II diabetes. More specifically, the process that takes place as a result of a high carbohydrate diet results in both obesity and diabetes. Oftentimes, losing 20 to 50 pounds (10 to 25 kilos) of body fat is all it takes to reverse or control Type II diabetes. Obesity interferes with normal glucose metabolism, and decreases insulin sensitivity. Insulin receptors on our fat storage cells don't work as well when these cells are "stuffed" with fat. Conversely, chronically high insulin levels make fat loss more difficult and may increase appetite.

You can develop Type II diabetes at any age if you are obese. In fact, diabetes

Exercise is beneficial in controlling, reversing, and preventing diabetes.

is increasing rapidly in children and young adults, because they eat so much and exercise so little.

Many people with diabetes avoid exercise. Inactivity combined with extra calories result in extra body pounds, which in turn makes diabetes worsen. More body fat and poorer blood sugar control then make exercising even more difficult. Yet exercise is one of the most powerful means to help prevent or control diabetes. Both anaerobic and aerobic exercise can permanently improve glucose metabolism, for the following reasons:

1. Exercise increases the metabolic rate and, with this increase, insulin receptors in muscle cells are activated. Glucose uptake is greatly enhanced over sedentary (sitting on the couch) levels.

2. With regular exercise, the body adapts to the training condition and uses insulin more efficiently. Japanese soldiers who were very active in their thirties were found to have less diabetes in their fifties. Men and women who make vigorous exercise a life-long habit rarely develop diabetes.

3. Regular exercise can increase insulin binding and receptor number, thus improving the uptake of glucose regardless of whether the body is exercising or at rest.

4. Regular exercise helps us lose body fat and not gain it back.
   a. Exercise can lower total and LDL cholesterol levels, decrease blood pressure, and improve circulation.
   b. Weight training exercise increases muscle mass. Muscles require plenty of glucose, but fat cells do not.

Thin People Can Be Diabetic, Too

What's really important is having a high ratio of lean to fat tissue in your total body weight. A high lean to fat ratio is associated with a strongly decreased risk for Type II diabetes. Lean tissue includes muscles, bones, tendons, ligaments, cartilage, and essential organs. Three hundred-pound body builders don't have diabetes because they have extra muscle, not extra fat. Muscles are the biggest users of glucose in your body. The more muscles you have (and the more you use them), the lower your risk for diabetes.

The lean to fat ratio is important even if you don't appear to be overweight. There's a big difference between being lean and being skinny. "Lean" means having a high ratio of lean to fat tissue. "Skinny" means you may not have too much body fat, but you don't have too much muscle, either! Skinny people have a lean to fat ratio that is average or even below average. Being skinny may be preferable to being obese, but it does not protect you from diabetes as much as being lean does.

Treatment and Prevention
with Supplements . . . .

There's good evidence that vitamin supplementation helps diabetes. Some vitamins help by directly lowering blood sugar. And in the long haul, a supplement plan represents excellent defense against developing diabetic complications.

A daily multivitamin is certainly helpful, but think of it only as the foundation of your nutrition program, not the entire program. "One-a-day" supplements with only recommended daily allowance (RDA) levels of nutrients are not enough to treat diabetes! You will need to supplement vitamins, antioxidants, trace elements, and some vitamin-like compounds. One pill can't do it alone. I'll explain which ones are the most important, so that you can minimize your pill intake as your lifestyle and budget dictate.

B Vitamins

B vitamins are vital for us to utilize glucose for energy. That's why white bread is bad for us–the B vitamins required for proper digestion and utilization of glucose are removed during the processing of white bread and other refined products. We can't fuel our bodies without B vitamins, and we are best off when they are supplemented all together. A multivitamin that provides 30 to 60 mg of each B vitamin in the B complex, 60 to 300 mcg of vitamin B_{12}, and 400 to 800 mcg of folic acid per day is recommended. Your multivitamin choice should also contain choline, inositol and PABA, at around 30 to 60 mg, and biotin at around 30 to 60 mcg (all in the B vitamin family).

In particular, Vitamin B_3 is essential for glucose metabolism. (Nicotinate, niacin, nicotinic acid, and nicotinamide are all names for vitamin B_3.) One of the symptoms of gross B_3 deficiency is a diabetic-like condition. As we'll discuss later on, chromium deficiency can also cause diabetic symptoms. Research has shown that chromium is not effective if B_3 is deficient, and vice versa

B_3 has also been used at 500 to 2,000 mg per day levels to slow the progression of Type I diabetes and fairly severe Type II diabetes with complications–but this manner of supplementation should be done under professional care only.

Vitamin B_6 deficiency is also clearly related to symptoms of

B vitamins are required for proper digestion and for utilization of glucose.

diabetes. The active form of B6, known as "pyridoxal phosphate," is absolutely required for the proper metabolism of carbohydrates. Vitamin B6 deficiency can cause high blood sugar, abnormal glucose tolerance, reduced insulin secretion, degeneration of the pancreatic cells that produce insulin and reduced insulin sensitivity. At least 30 mg B6 per day should be taken to prevent diabetes, and 40 to 100 mg per day are recommended for treating existing Type I and Type II diabetes. Don't just supplement B6 alone–"piggy back" extra B6 onto your multivitamin.

The combination of Vitamin B6, folic acid, and vitamin B12 are crucial for you, because these vitamins work together to prevent the excessive accumulation of homocysteine in the body. Homocysteine is a natural biochemical product of our metabolism, but levels that are too high increase your risk for heart disease, blocked arteries, and small blood vessel disorders.

Antioxidants

Antioxidants are a must for preventing diabetic complications, and may directly improve glucose tolerance and insulin sensitivity. Antioxidants include vitamin C, vitamin E, vitamin A, beta-carotene, selenium, zinc, and herbal products such as grape seed, pine bark, green tea, rosemary, and curcumin. Antioxidants are

Almost all diabetics can benefit from taking extra vitamin C.

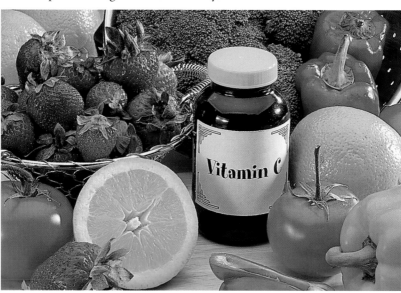

synergistic, meaning they work best when supplemented in combination. Combined antioxidant supplementation has been shown to reduce the increased risk of heart disease associated with diabetes.

Antioxidants	
• alpha-lipoic acid	• green tea
• bilberry	• pine bark extract (pycnogenol)
• coenzyme Q-10	• selenium
• cysteine	• vitamin A and beta-carotene
• ginkgo biloba	• vitamin C
• glutathione	• vitamin E
• grape seed extract	• zinc

Antioxidants are generally beneficial because diabetics typically have higher levels of oxidative stress than do nondiabetics. Recall our discussion of "protein glycation," excess blood glucose bonding with hemoglobin and other proteins in the bloodstream and tissues. If blood sugar is chronically elevated, the daily effort needed to "clean up" the compounds formed by protein glycation is believed to overwhelm the body's detoxification systems, leading to chronically higher oxidative stress.

Vitamin C uptake by cells in the body is promoted by insulin, and it's inhibited by high blood sugar. Consequently, Type I diabetics in particular may be chronically deficient in C, and may not be able to utilize C as efficiently as healthy people can. A six-year study of more than 2,000 diabetic and nondiabetic persons found that blood vitamin C levels were lower in those with newly diagnosed diabetes than in nondiabetics.

Almost all diabetics can benefit greatly from vitamin C supplementation in excess of RDA levels. Supplementing with 500 mg per day is quite safe. This can improve performance on glucose tolerance tests, and can reduce the insulin requirement for insulin-dependent diabetics. In a study of 241 humans, lower blood levels of vitamin C were correlated with higher levels of fasting blood sugar. In another study, patients visiting a clinic were given 500 mg vitamin C twice per day for ten days, and glucose tolerance improved in all patients.

Diabetics appear to have a greater need for L-carnitine than most people.

Vitamin E can improve glucose tolerance and reduce insulin requirements.

Vitamin E is synergistic with C, and can further improve glucose tolerance test performance while also reducing insulin requirements.

In one study, 900 mg (not IU) vitamin E per day were given to fifteen Type II patients and ten normal controls for four months. Glucose metabolism and tolerance were improved in both diabetic and normal subjects; however, the researchers did not advocate such high levels of supplementation without longer-term studies. In various studies, vitamin E supplementation ranging from 400 to 1,800 international units (IU) per day has greatly reduced risk factors for diabetic complications.

Alpha-lipoic acid is not a vitamin; rather, it is a fat-soluble antioxidant, and an enzyme co-factor used in energy metabolism. It is best supplemented, but is found naturally in foods like spinach and potatoes. It may directly lower blood sugar by improving the utilization of glucose. Alpha-lipoic acid given at 500 mg intravenously for fourteen days was shown to improve glucose utilization by 20 to 50 percent; meanwhile, a similar study with 600 mg by mouth for 30 days showed less spectacular results. I'd recommend taking alpha-lipoic acid at 200 to 600 mg per day for at least three months to see improvements.

The term "antioxidant" includes vitamins, minerals, and herbal products. More detailed information about zinc and selenium will be discussed later on. Here's a basic list to both treat and prevent diabetes. Note that diabetics may have difficulty converting beta-carotene to vitamin A, so they are best off supplementing both.

Suggested Antioxidant Supplementation (per day)

1,000 mg vitamin C with bioflavonoids 3 to 4 times per day
8,000 IU vitamin A
20,000 IU beta-carotene
100 to 200 mcg selenium, as selenomethionine
20 mg zinc, amino acid chelated
800 IU vitamin E, preferably as mixed natural tocopherols
200 to 600 mg alpha-lipoic acid

Please Note: If you have diabetic kidney disease or other kidney dysfunction, please consult your physician before supplementing more than 1,000 mg C three times per day (3,000 mg total).

Vitamin D deficiency has been linked to glucose intolerance in the elderly. In a research study, fourteen Dutch men aged 70 to 88 had their vitamin D levels tested. Thirty-nine percent were vitamin D deficient, and those with lower vitamin D levels performed worse on glucose tolerance tests and had higher levels of insulin.

Lack of vitamin D is already considered a major cause of chronic infections, weak bones and muscles, and heart disease in older persons. It's estimated that currently 30 to 50 percent of the elderly are vitamin D deficient! At the other end of the spectrum, vitamin D supplementation in infancy is associated with a reduced risk for Type I diabetes. Vitamin D is crucial for immunity, and it's thought that having adequate vitamin D helps prevent the immune system dysregulation that enables pancreatic beta-cells to be attacked.

Vitamin D differs from all other essential nutrients in that humans are capable of manufacturing all they need with only 20 to 30 minutes of sun exposure on the skin three to five days per week.

Only 400 to 600 IU vitamin D in your multivitamin is sufficient. Rely more heavily on regular, brief sunlight exposure. Sunlight is much safer than high levels of supplementation, which must be administered under professional care.

L-carnitine can help insulin work better; it helps to normalize the high levels of insulin that Type II diabetics often have. L-carnitine is also required for the body to burn stored fat, so it may aid in weight loss as well as in lowering cholesterol and triglycerides. Diabetics appear have a greater need for L-carnitine, yet, paradoxically, they excrete L-carnitine at a greater rate than do nondiabetic persons.

L-carnitine is found naturally only in animal protein foods–especially in raw or rare meat. It can be made by the body from L-lysine; however, not everybody makes amounts that are optimum for good health. Our modern diets–especially vegetarian diets–provide little or no L-carnitine compared with the diets of modern traditional hunting societies, or with the diets that our paleolithic ancestors are believed to have eaten.

Anyone who wishes to prevent or treat diabetes might want to consider taking 1 to 2 grams L-carnitine per day. For treatment

Diabetics appear to have a greater need for L-carnitine than most people.

of active diabetes, 1.5 to 3 grams are recommended. Please note that at this time L-carnitine is not legally sold in Canada due to nonsensical regulations.

Gestational Diabetes

Gestational diabetes, which develops during pregnancy, is much more similar to Type II than it is to Type I diabetes. It's more common in Hispanics, Native Americans, Asians, and African-Americans than it is in Caucasians.

It's also more common in older and overweight mothers. To prevent or treat gestational diabetes, exercise throughout pregnancy, don't gain more than 24 to 30 pounds (12 to 15 kilos), and take your prenatal vitamins.

In addition, you can safely supplement 50 to 100 mg B6, 800 mcg chromium picolinate, and 400 to 600 mg magnesium per day if you are at risk for gestational diabetes.

B6 is of special concern for women, since it's required for regulating the menstrual cycle, pregnancy, and nursing. Later in the term of a pregnancy, women may experience leg muscle cramps, carpal tunnel syndrome, irritability, fluid retention and gestational diabetes. All of these conditions are related to vitamin B6 deficiency induced by pregnancy, and can be alleviated by supplementing 40 to 100 mg B6 per day.

The diet we discussed earlier (see page 14) is an excellent diet for gestational diabetes, and it provides good, overall nutrition principles for pregnant women.

After the child is born, you can help prevent diabetes in yourself–and in your child later in life–by breastfeeding for at least six months. To further reduce the risk to your child, avoid feeding wheat, rye, cow's milk, peanuts, and soybeans (except soy formula as medically prescribed) for 12 months. Instead feed your child whole foods such as puréed carrots and apples.

The mineral chromium is required for normal insulin functioning.

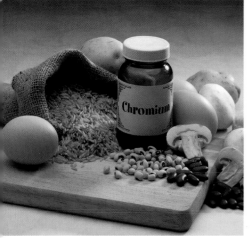

Chromium

Chromium is an essential trace element, required for normal insulin functioning, It is also the single most important trace element for diabetics to supplement. Chromium deficiency produces diabetic symptoms, including high blood sugar, unstable blood sugar and reduced insulin sensitivity. Lack of chromium also causes increased total cholesterol and triglycerides, but decreased HDL ("good") cholesterol.

It is generally believed that many years of consuming a diet that's low in chromium will eventually "catch up" to people as they reach middle age; we also tend to excrete more chromium in the urine as we age. Both of these factors may contribute to the development of Type II diabetes.

Chromium in Foods

According to the US Department of Agriculture, 90 percent of Americans don't obtain the estimated safe and adequate daily dietary intake (ESADSI) of 50 to 200 mcg per day of chromium (there's no RDA established yet). Similar widespread deficiencies have also been documented in Canada, Britain, and Finland.

Brewer's yeast, beer, whole grains, cheese, liver, and other meats can be good dietary sources of chromium; however, chromium content varies widely in foods. The refining of flour and sugars and the processing of foods removes most of their absorbable chromium content.

High consumption of sugars and refined carbohydrates increases chromium excretion in the urine by 10 to 300 percent; consequently, we have no option other than to supplement if we want to prevent and treat diabetes throughout the population of Western countries.

Supplementing chromium: The chromium supplement that is currently on the market, and which has been shown to be the most effective and best absorbed, is chromium picolinate. Chromium is also sold as chromium citrate, and is chelated with amino acids such as arginine and glycine, all of which are acceptable supplements. Chromium chloride is not recommended; and chromium nicotinate complexes are not stable.

Chromium supplementation at 200 to 400 mcg per day helps to prevent Type II diabetes. But doses of 1,000 to 1,200 mcg per day are recommended for treating existing diabetes.

A 1997 controlled study of Type II diabetics compared low doses, high doses, and no doses (placebo) of chromium. Sixty patients received 500 mcg chromium picolinate twice per day for four months, which lowered fasting blood glucose, post-meal blood glucose, and nearly normalized glycated hemoglobin levels compared with the 60 patients who received the placebo. Total cholesterol and insulin levels also dropped with the 1,000 mcg dose. A third group of 60 received 100 mcg chromium twice per day, which somewhat lowered glycated hemoglobin and insulin levels, but blood glucose was not lowered.

A 1999 controlled study also showed that 1,000 mcg chromium picolinate per day for eight months significantly improved insulin sensitivity in 29 Type II diabetics.

If you have Type II diabetes and are taking medication to control your blood sugar, start with 200 mcg chromium per day for a week, and monitor your glucose closely. Increase by 200 mcg per week until you reach 1,000 to 1,200 mcg, and then, since you won't need as much of the drug, have your doctor adjust your medication accordingly.

For Type I diabetes, use the same approach: Add chromium in 100 to 200 mcg increments per week. Monitor your glucose closely, because you should experience a decrease in your insulin requirements. If you have trouble adjusting the insulin dose you take just before going to bed, do not take chromium supplements within three hours of retiring. Work up to the level of chromium that allows you to consistently reduce your daytime insulin, and stabilize your insulin requirements. Then work on the night dosage.

Magnesium

This mineral is needed to transport glucose to our cells, and to regulate how we use food to produce energy. Magnesium is required for the production and release of insulin; it is also required by cells for normal insulin sensitivity and receptor number.

Our glucose metabolism can't function normally if magnesium is deficient. Unfortunately, magnesium levels are often depleted in diabetics, especially Type I diabetics. Apparently, diabetes results in a higher requirement for magnesium–but, unfortunately, it results in a higher rate of magnesium excretion in the urine as well.

Magnesium is also a major trace element component of our bones, and helps to normalize blood pressure. It's needed for proper muscle and nerve function, and plays a role in regulating one's heartbeat. In a nutshell, magnesium is critical to our health, and we simply can't live very long with a severe magnesium deficiency. If the deficiency is not severe but our magnesium levels are still suboptimal, we may remain alive, but we exist as "walking wounded."

Magnesium in foods: Fresh vegetables (especially green vegetables) and fruits are the best foods for getting magnesium in your diet. Significant amounts of magnesium are lost, however, during the course of food processing and cooking. (When green vegetables take on a grayish caste from overcooking, this indicates that the magnesium has been lost from the vegetables.) Higher amounts of magnesium are found in raw and lightly steamed fruits and vegetables.

Meat, fish, shellfish, nuts, and dairy products are also good food sources of magnesium. A diet that's high in sugars, refined flours and/or alcohol will not meet the daily magnesium requirements for a healthy person, and such a diet is definitely not optimal for a person with diabetes.

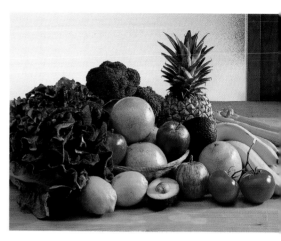

Fresh fruit and vegetables provide magnesium in the diet.

Supplementing magnesium: In addition to making an effort to eat magnesium-rich foods, it's beneficial for Type II and gestational diabetics to supplement 400 to 800 mg of magnesium per day. Unlike many other minerals, magnesium is fairly well absorbed in a variety of forms, so magnesium oxide, magnesium hydroxide, and magnesium carbonate are fine to use. Magnesium citrate, magnesium aspartate and magnesium lactate are better absorbed than oxides or carbonates, but you will have to take more pills per day as these sources are not as concentrated.

Dolomite and oyster shell are not recommended as magnesium or calcium supplements as they are not from an organic source such as spinach or sardines.

Please Note: If you have Type I diabetes, diabetic kidney disease, or other kidney dysfunction, please consult your physician before supplementing magnesium. Magnesium supplementation may not be beneficial for people whose excretion of trace element salts is impaired. If you have these conditions, it is best to stick only to consuming a diet that's sufficient in magnesium.

Zinc

People with diabetes tend to have zinc levels that are lower than optimal. This is an important point for diabetics, because zinc is involved in thousands of bodily functions. Most importantly, zinc is considered to be an antioxidant trace element because it's a component of many of the enzymes that our bodies use to neutralize toxic substances. In addition, our skin, hair, nails, bones, liver, mental acuity, senses, fat metabolism, circulatory, reproductive, and immune systems require zinc, and they break down rapidly when it's lacking. All new tissue growth, eyesight, taste and smell, athletic performance, and dental health require zinc.

There is general agreement among nutrition scientists that moderate, but not excessive, zinc supplementation will improve the overall health of diabetics, with very little cost or risk. There is no consensus, however, regarding whether or not zinc supplementation can result in significant improvements in blood sugar control. In some cases, supplemental zinc has improved performance on glucose tolerance tests, but those who were taking these tests may have been grossly deficient in zinc.

Zinc in foods: Zinc from animal proteins is more absorbable than zinc obtained from other sources. Oysters are among the richest sources of zinc. Lean red meat has twice as much zinc as does white meat such as poultry but, in general, meat and fish are the major sources of zinc in the diet. Vegetarians may get zinc from eating brewer's yeast, dulse, egg yolks, kelp, mushrooms, pecans, soybenas, sunflower seeds, and soy lecithin. Dairy products, grains, and legumes provide much less.

Supplementing zinc: If your multivitamin choice has 25 to 30 mg per day, this is sufficient. If the levels are lower, take a 20 to 30 mg zinc supplement every other day. Zinc picolinate, gluconate, aspartate, monomethionine, and other amino acid chelated products are good choices for zinc supplements. Avoid zinc oxide, and especially zinc sulfate, which can cause nausea for a short time after you take it.

Other Important Minerals

Selenium, manganese, copper, and calcium are also important nutrients in terms of diabetes. Selenium is an antioxidant, and it's best to supplement antioxidants as a group. Recommended supplementation is 100 to 200 mcg selenium as selenomethionine.

Gross deficiencies of manganese and copper may cause or contribute to abnormally high blood sugar, but supplementing these minerals beyond normal requirements doesn't provide additional benefits. Diets that feature meat, fish, shellfish, nuts, and fresh fruits and vegetables generally provide enough manganese and copper. In addition, many multivitamins provide about 5 to

7 mg manganese and 2 to 3 mg copper, which are safe and sufficient levels of supplementation.

More severe cases of diabetes may be associated with abnormal calcium metabolism, but this may be a consequence rather than a cause of diabetes. Calcium is deficient in many diets, especially if dairy products, sardines and herring are not eaten. Claims that tofu, soy milk, beans, broccoli, whole grains, and collard greens can provide enough calcium in the diet are exaggerated. Most people don't eat collards daily, for example–and try feeding them to a toddler! Calcium is also absorbed better from dairy products than from soy food, beans, and grains.

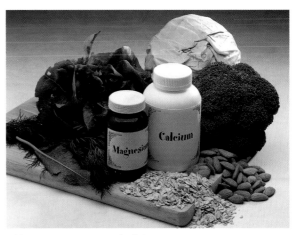

Calcium and magnesium are best supplemented together for more effective absorption.

Magnesium and calcium need to work together, so it's best to supplement 400 to 800 mg calcium along with magnesium, but only if your diet doesn't supply much calcium.

Please Note: If you have Type I diabetes, diabetic kidney disease or other kidney dysfunction, please consult your physician before supplementing calcium. Calcium supplementation may not be beneficial for people whose excretion of trace element salts is impaired. If you have these conditions, it is best to stick only to consuming a diet that's sufficient in calcium.

Food allergies, especially to wheat and other glutenous grains, can cause reduced absorption of calcium and other trace elements. Don't rely on dairy, soy or other legumes as a source of calcium if you know or suspect you're allergic to them.

Treatment and Prevention with Herbs and Nutraceuticals . . . .

Plant foods and herbs play a larger role in blood sugar control than most people realize. Hundreds of research studies have come to the same conclusion: The higher one's consumption of fruits and vegetables in the diet, the lower one's risk will be for any chronic disease, from cancer to diabetes. Conversely, the people in these many studies who ate few fruits and vegetables were more prone to disease, and more likely to die prematurely. This is thought to be due to the vitamins, minerals, fiber, and beneficial phytochemicals which fruits and vegetables contain. ("Phytochemical" means a naturally occurring chemical made by a plant.)

Many plant foods today, however, are much poorer sources of the phytochemicals and fiber that have the potential to help diabetes, compared with the plant foods our ancestors consumed. In fact, our ancestors' diets were exceedingly rich in phytochemicals compared to our diets today, and we have come to realize that humans literally evolved bathed in these phytochemicals. It is likely that we are adapted to having these compounds in our diet; it is equally likely that keeping our blood sugar normal depends in part on their presence.

Luckily, there's an easy solution here–and you don't have to go graze in your yard for weeds! Certainly you do need to eat plenty of vegetables. But there are herbal and functional food products available that have proven to be effective in terms of diabetes. These products provide the "missing" phytochemicals and fiber in an easy, concentrated, and digestible form. These products are available in your quality health food stores.

Literally hundreds of medicinal and culinary plants have been shown to directly lower blood sugar, but few of these plants have been investigated in detail. In the next two sections we discuss plants that have proven themselves in controlled human studies to be safe and effective for lowering blood sugar. Herbal products alone can't be expected to control or reverse diabetes, of course, but they are helpful when used in conjunction with other approaches. Follow the manufacturer's dosage recommendations on the label for guidance.

Medicinal Plants

Korean ginseng (Panax ginseng) has been used for diabetes in traditional Chinese medicine for centuries. On the Western side of the planet, a 1995 Finnish study found that 200 mg ginseng per day for eight weeks lowered fasting blood

Ginseng is a traditional Chinese remedy for diabetes.

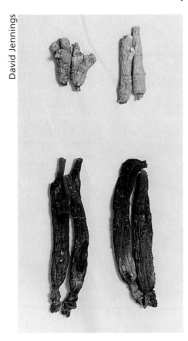

David Jennings

glucose and body weight compared to placebo. The people in the study who received ginseng also reported that their mood improved and they were more physically active. The ginseng dosage used in this study wasn't very large by the standards of most herbal experts, since it comprised just one capsule. A more appropriate dosage would be four capsules per day.

Type I diabetics and Type II diabetics taking antidiabetic medications should start with one capsule and increase by one capsule per week. Monitor your blood sugar closely, but don't expect dramatic changes like you'd see from chromium.

Gurmar (Gymnena sylvestre) is an ancient Indian treatment for diabetes, which has proven effective in some recent studies when taken for at least six months. It is believed that gurmar stimulates insulin secretion–so it may not be appropriate for people with chronically high levels of circulating insulin. This would include most people with Type II diabetes, but nobody with Type I diabetes.

Gurmar does not seem to lower blood sugar levels in all people, and may take a few months to show positive results. It's worth a try, however, because it has also been shown to lower cholesterol and triglycerides without side effects.

One capsule of a standardized extract can be taken two to four times per day. Type I diabetics, or Type II diabetics using antidiabetic medications, should start with one capsule per day and increase by one capsule per week for four weeks, monitoring blood sugar closely.

Fig leaf (Ficus carica) and ivy gourd leaf (coccinia indica) aren't normally available in the North American market, but they, or similar leaves, will perhaps become available in the future. In a Spanish study of Type I diabetics, one cup of unsweetened fig leaf tea taken with breakfast for a month lowered insulin requirements by 12 percent. In a Pakistani study, six tablets of ivy gourd leaves per day for six weeks decreased fasting glucose and improved glucose tolerance in Type II diabetics by 20 percent.

Milk thistle (Silybum marianum) is primarily known as an antioxidant and liver protectant. It's not considered to lower blood sugar in otherwise healthy Type II diabetics, but could be very useful for Type I diabetics, and any diabetic with liver disease or dysfunction.

Gurmar is an ancient Indian remedy for diabetes.

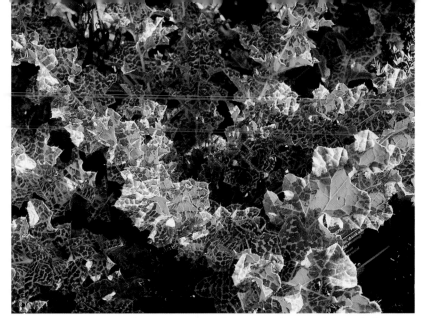

Milk thistle is beneficial for Type I diabetics, and any diabetic with liver disease.

In animal studies, a condition similar to Type I diabetes is induced by damaging the beta cells of the pancreas with drugs. Several related phytochemicals (known as silymarin) from milk thistle have consistently reduced damage done to the pancreas by the drugs, but silymarin needs to be given along with the drugs or shortly afterwards. Upon a new diagnosis of Type I diabetes, it makes sense to start on milk thistle to help prevent further damage to the pancreas.

Silymarin has also been shown to reduce diabetic nerve damage in humans and animals. The liver handles most of the storage and release of glycogen, so if liver function is compromised, insulin resistance and diabetes in general is more severe. In an Italian study, 30 insulin-dependent Type II diabetics with liver cirrhosis (due to alcoholism) were given 600 mg silymarin per day, and 30 others were not. Both groups got standard therapy for their condition. After four months, the 30 diabetics receiving silymarin reduced their fasting insulin levels and required insulin dosage, while the 30 others did not.

Please Note: Achieving the dosages used in these studies requires a high-quality, standardized milk thistle product. For long-term use, 200 to 300 mg silymarin (may also be listed as silybin) per day is recommended. Do not use milk thistle without consulting a professional if you have known or suspected liver disease or are taking any medications.

Nutraceuticals and Culinary Herbs

Bitter melon (Momordica charantia) is used traditionally in India, Africa, and Asia as a diabetic remedy and as a "bitter tonic" food. It's available fresh in most Asian groceries. Regular use of bitter melon has been shown to lower blood sugar, sugar in the urine, and glycated hemoglobin, both gradually and cumulatively.

Fresh bitter melon juices or decoctions are considered to be the most effective preparations. A decoction is made by pouring boiling water over chopped fresh fruit, steeping and then straining.

To use bitter melon, eat cooked sliced bitter melon with one to two meals per day, or drink the decocted juice as described above. You may need to start with only a few slices or 50 ml juice and work up to 200 ml after three weeks. Use 200 ml for four weeks, and monitor your progress. Then adjust your intake downward to an effective maintenance dosage. Use this gradual approach for Type I treatment also.

Standardized encapsulated bitter melon extract is becoming available, providing a more convenient alternative. Follow the manufacturer's recommended dosage, which will be around three to six capsules per day.

Holy basil (Ocimum sanctum) is used in India and Southeast Asia as a food and medicinal plant. Holy basil has an anise-like taste, and is a common flavor in Thai cuisine. In an Indian study, patients were given one gram of dried holy basil leaf per day for 30 days. This lowered their fasting blood glucose by 21 percent, and also lowered glycated hemoglobin, total cholesterol, LDL ("bad") cholesterol and triglycerides.

While these results are encouraging, more research is needed, because the patients in this study also continued taking their antidiabetic medications throughout the course of the study. This means that basil may have just acted to help the medication work, or that much higher doses of holy basil would be needed to treat diabetes without the medication.

In the meantime, since holy basil is a food plant, it's safe to use 1 to 3 grams of the dried powdered herb per day. Note that all varieties of basil, mint, oregano, thyme, sage, savory, and rosemary are members of the mint family of plants. Mint family plants are rich in antioxidants, and as such they're used medicinally

Bitter melon is a traditional remedy, and is used in India, Africa, and Asia.

37

all over the world. It's a good idea to use them liberally in your cooking, and/or drink herbal teas containing these herbs.

Onions (Allium cepa) and garlic (Allium sativum) both have sulfur-containing phytochemicals, which may improve insulin's effectiveness. One of these sulfur phytochemicals is called alliin. In a 1992 German study, 800 mg per day of garlic standardized for its alliin content was given for four weeks. Those receiving garlic lowered their fasting blood glucose, while those receiving placebo did not. In another study, garlic powder with no alliin was given at 700 mg per day for four weeks, but had no effect.

Other research concludes that only massive amounts of onions and garlic could be helpful. Onions and garlic should be used in addition to other herbal and nutritional treatments. It's good practice to eat onions, garlic, leeks, shallots or chives on a daily basis. Raw would be your first choice, then very lightly cooked. Otherwise, take 3 to 8 standardized garlic capsules/tablets per day.

Garlic is also an antioxidant, lowers cholesterol, and may improve intermittent claudication (a complication of diabetes), so it is generally beneficial for diabetics.

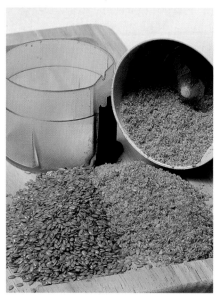

Flaxseeds can be easily ground in an electric coffee grinder.

38

Flaxseed (Linum usitatissimum) is one of the richest sources of fiber known, containing both soluble and insoluble fiber. In a University of Toronto study, people ate either plain white bread or bread with 25 percent flaxseed meal. The flaxseed bread improved glucose tolerance by 28 percent compared to the white bread.

They were also given water with flaxseed mucilage (a soluble fiber extracted from the flaxseeds), or plain water. The mucilage drink improved glucose tolerance by 27 percent compared with plain water. Mucilage can act to inhibit glucose absorption, but the mucilage content of flaxseed is only a few percent. Since the flaxseed meal bread worked just as well, it's thought that protein, fats, and phytochemicals in flaxseed work synergistically with the fiber content to lower blood sugar.

The best way to use flaxseed is to purchase flaxseeds and grind them in an electric coffee grinder. This process is inexpensive and allows you to grind only what you need so there's no risk of eating rancid oils from the mixture. Three to nine teaspoons of ground flaxseed can be used per day with no gastrointestinal discomfort. For both Type I and Type II diabetes, start with one teaspoon flax twice per day and increase to three teaspoons twice per day. Make sure you mix the flaxseed with water or another liquid; do not consume it dry.

Fenugreek (Trigonella foenum-graecum) is a traditional Indian remedy for diabetes and heart disease. Whole fenugreek seeds are 50 percent fiber, with 20 percent of that mucilage.

In an Indian study, Type I diabetic patients were given either meals with 100 grams of defatted ground fenugreek seeds per day, or regular meals. After ten days, fasting glucose decreased by 30 percent and glucose tolerance improved in those who consumed fenugreek.

In other studies, 15 to 25 grams of fenugreek powder were similarly effective for Type II diabetics, and five gram doses may help prevent mild cases of diabetes from worsening. In all studies, fenugreek was found very effective in lowering LDL ("bad") cholesterol and triglycerides.

Powdered fenugreek is available in bulk from Indian groceries or spice suppliers. Start with one-fourth teaspoon stirred in a glass of water three times per day, and increase to a heaping teaspoon three or four times per day. One drawback is that fenugreek at these levels will almost certainly cause flatulence. If this bothers you, lower your dosage and combine fenugreek with other herbs. Alternatively, look for standardized defatted fenugreek fiber. This product is designed to be effective at 5 to 10 gram doses.

Prickly pear (Nopal) cactus (Opuntia spp.) is widely used as a food throughout Latin America. Nopal is rich in pectin, a type of soluble fiber.

Flaxseed, an excellent source of fiber, improves glucose tolerance.

In a Mexican hospital study, diabetics were given 500 grams of either fresh cooked or raw nopal on an empty stomach. After 180 minutes, fasting glucose was lowered 22 to 25 percent by cooked or raw nopal, as compared to 6 percent for water. Since fasting glucose was lowered in this study, it's apparent that there's synergistic benefits from nopal, too.

To use nopal, purchase the fresh cactus from a grocery that has a Latin American produce section. Eat 1 to 2 cups cooked or raw every day. Canned nopal and nopal salsas are also widely available. Preparations from dried pieces of cactus have not been shown conclusively to be effective. Encapsulated nopal products are available; follow the manufacturer's suggested dosage on the label.

Antioxidant-Rich Herbs

As part of your antioxidant supplementation, I'd suggest picking some of the following to use daily, or look for a blended botanical antioxidant at your health food store. Feel free to experiment–rotate or alternate products, buy what's on sale, etc.

• Any "green drink"–many labels state that they contain botanical antioxidants. Drink 1 to 3 servings per day, depending on your produce intake.

• In addition to or instead of a green drink, take 2 to 4 capsules/tablets of any of the following per day. Pick up to four individual products, but if you want to use only one, curcumin is the one to choose. Curcumin is known to specifically reduce hemoglobin glycation and cross-linking of collagen, the protein that comprises a majority of our connective tissue. (Connective tissue includes skin, blood vessel walls, tendons, ligaments, cartilage, and bone organic matrix.)

• bee propolis
• cayenne
• curcumin
• garlic
• grape seed extract
• green tea beverage or extract
• licorice
• milk thistle
• mixed bioflavonoids (i.e., rutin, quercetin, citrus peel extract)
• mixed natural carotenoids
• oregano, thyme, peppermint, spearmint, or other mint family plants, preferably as herbal teas
• pine bark extract (i.e., Pycnogenol®)
• rosemary extract
• schizandra
• Siberian ginseng

Many plants traditionally used to treat diabetes around the world have been investigated in laboratory animals and in cell cultures.

In Canada, a tea blend of many promising herbs (Eleotin) has lowered blood sugar in preliminary human and animal trials. One important herb in this blend is schizandra, an antioxidant herb that is known to shorten post-exercise recovery time by improving liver function and storage of glycogen.

In Japan and the US, an extract of Lagerstrotroemia speciosa (glucosol), whose active ingredient is the phytochemical corosolic acid, has dramatically lowered blood sugar in preliminary human studies.

Eleotin

About 25 years ago a woman suffering from serious diabetes and kidney disease decided to spend her final days travelling, opting against the amputation her doctors recommended. She was told she would eventually die without the operation. While on a trip to Asia she was offered many traditional folk remedies, herbal medicines, and alternative treatments. With nothing to lose, she tried many of them. After several months she began to feel stronger and had a renewed sense of peace and appreciation for life.

Upon her return her doctor ran a complete set of test and was surprised to find that both her diabetes and kidney disease had improved and she no longer required amputation to save her life. Astonished by this turnaround, doctors decided to direct a research team to trace the footsteps of her trip in detail. The traditional, medicinal herbs that were learned of, which are regarded as restorative agents, became the starting point for a safe and natural supplement that enhances blood sugar control.

Almost two decades later, this specially formulated herbal blend is a safe health food that restores the body's own ability to control blood glucose levels. It is a promising herbal treatment for lowering blood glucose levels for Type II diabetics. Various dried roots, stems, fruits, and leaves are made into a tea form.

In China and the US, an extract of He Shou Wu (fo ti; polygonum multiflorum) has been patented for the treatment of diabetes, proving effective in Chinese clinical trials both on its own and in combination with cinnamon and chromium.

At the US Department of Agriculture in Beltsville, Maryland, more than 60 plants have been investigated, with findings indicating that an extract from cinnamon was by far the most

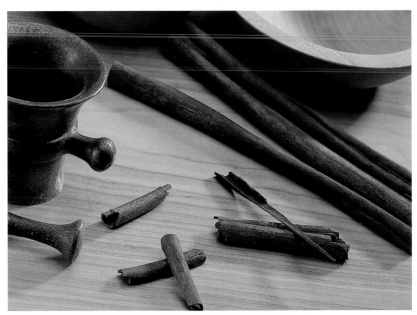

There are many herbal remedies and combinations, either on the market or still in the research stages, to treat diabetes.

effective at helping cells use glucose. The cinnamon extract is also an antioxidant. I've heard from hundreds of people who have successfully used cinnamon to lower their blood sugar and/or insulin requirements. Since cinnamon is very safe and tasty, there's little harm in trying it yourself.

To use cinnamon, put three rounded tablespoons ground cinnamon and 1 teaspoon baking soda in a quart canning jar. Fill the jar with boiling water, and allow it to steep at room temperature until cool. Strain off the liquid and discard the "grounds," then cover the jar and refrigerate. Drink 1 cup (240 ml; 8 oz.) of the tea four times per day. After three weeks, drop to 2 to 4 cups per day, or use as needed. Give children half doses in the same manner. For people with Type I diabetes, or those using antidiabetic medications, start with 1 to 2 cups per day, and increase by one cup per week, monitoring blood sugar closely.

Conclusion . . . .

Put simply, your nutrition and lifestyle choices dictate whether or not you have Type II diabetes. Type II diabetes is anything but a high-tech disease. It's a low-tech disease brought on by straying from the diet and lifestyle that our bodies are geared for. In many ways the answer to Type II diabetes is low tech also, moving back in time to a high fiber, high protein diet, more omega-3 fats, medicinal plants and spices, pure water, and higher levels of many nutrients than processed grains and sugars can ever provide.

If you have Type I diabetes, you can use this book's information to lower your insulin dosages, and be "proactive" in preventing complications. Typical advice given to diabetics is "keep your blood sugar low and stable to help prevent complications." Period. This is good advice, but only scratches the surface of how you can prevent complications with antioxidants and herbs, for example.

The most important piece of advice I can give you from my heart is to set a good example. You can't nag your mother, father, husband, etc. to change their diets, exercise, and take vitamins if they are just not willing. But you can smile and go about doing it yourself, and if appropriate, for your children. And as you get healthier, there's a good chance those you'd like to help will come around to your way of thinking. Sometimes their motivation is only jealousy, but more often it will stem from love and respect, and a genuine desire to do whatever it takes to live a life free of diabetes.

If appeals to the heart and intellect haven't gotten to you, how about your wallet? Consider the taxpayer burden we all share: Diabetes cost US Medicare alone a staggering 42.5 billion dollars in 1995, and costs have increased every year since. The US Congress noticed this financial drain, and the 1999 budget had a line item mandating government research on chromium for diabetes.

Set a good example for your children by providing and eating healthful foods.

However, if you have diabetes, don't sit around being a government health statistic for the new millennium. There's no question that chromium as well as the other supplements and dietary advice we've discussed can help diabetes without dangerous side effects. You can start feeling better and saving money today.

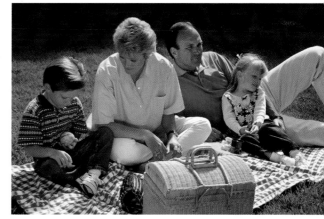

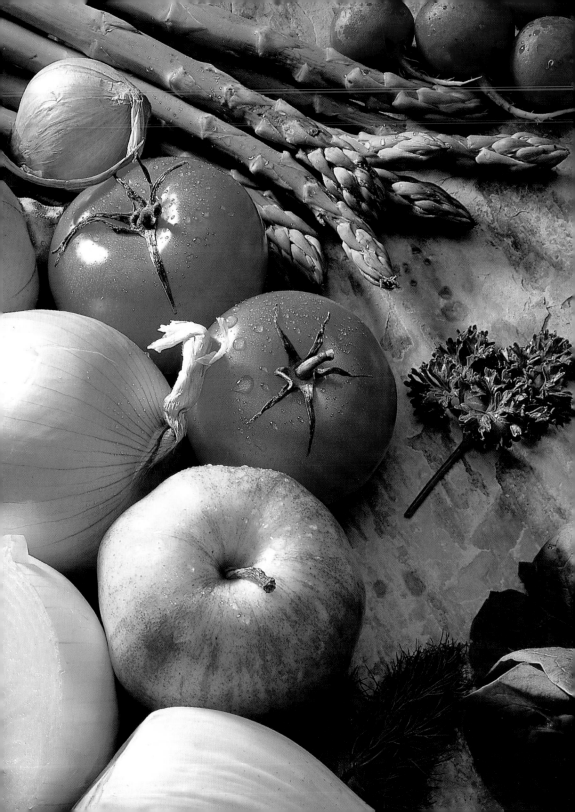

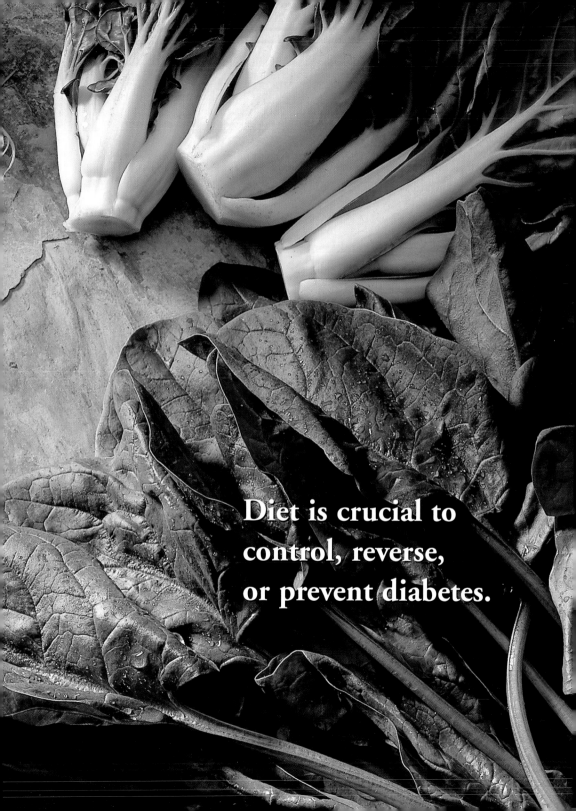

Diet is crucial to
control, reverse,
or prevent diabetes.

Best Blender Drink Ever

There is no substitute for the fluffy smooth texture that mango provides in this recipe, (although bananas or peaches are good choices as well) and it will give you the smoothest, fluffiest blender drink you've ever made. And if you choose to use whole milk, you'll never want to buy ice cream again! The technique here is similar to the way rich ice cream is made, but the blender drink is a much healthier alternative. An industrial-strength blender like Vita-mixer is vastly superior to a blender, and is a great investment if you plan to make blender drinks often.

1 large ripe mango,
   peeled and pitted

1 tbsp coconut oil, at
   room temperature

1 package tropical fruit,
   vanilla or strawberry
   flavored EAS Myoplex
   meal replacement powder
   (or equivalent
   brand such as Met-Rx)

½ tsp unpasteurized
   honey

⅛–¼ tsp sea salt

1 ¼ cups (310 ml) water
   or whole milk

12–24 ice cubes, to taste

Place mango, oil, meal replacement powder, salt, and sweetener in a blender. Add the water and blend until smooth, adding a bit more water if needed. You need to emulsify the coconut oil. Never add coconut oil after the ice, or it will freeze into a single lump!

Add 1 to 2 trays of ice, a few pieces at a time, and a dash of water as needed, and blend until smooth.

If there is too much to blend properly, pour out some "concentrate" into a glass before adding all the ice, then blend the rest with ice in two batches.

Variations: If you don't have coconut oil, use a generous tablespoon of soft (not melted) butter instead, following the same technique, although the drink will not come out quite as fluffy. You can also add 1 or 2 tablespoons of freshly ground flax seed meal, or 1 teaspoon of ground cinnamon.

Serves 1

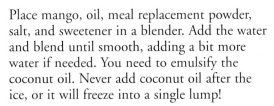

mango

Although the mango peels are bitter, they are filled with beneficial phytochemicals, so I eat the peels just for the nutrition while preparing the drink. Please don't put peels in the drink or you'll spoil the flavor and texture. Note also that ripe mangoes must be really soft. It can take weeks for them to ripen off the tree, so buy the ripest mangoes you can, and don't refrigerate until they are soft and fragrant.

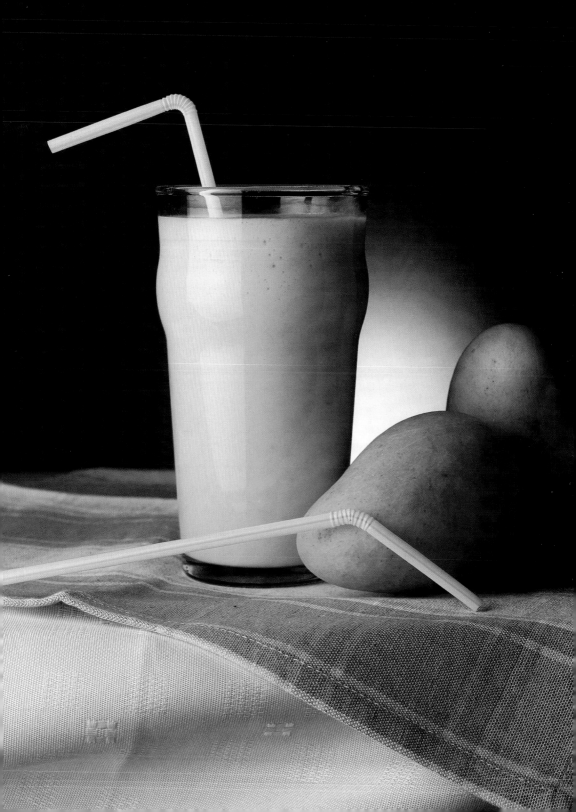

Tomato-Asparagus Fritatta

This nutritious and filling fritatta is wonderful any time of the day–breakfast, lunch, or dinner. Onions help lower blood sugar because of their active ingredients allyl propyl disulphide (APDS) and diallyl disulphide oxide (allicin).

¼ cup (60 ml) **red bell pepper, finely chopped**

¼ cup (60 ml) **yellow bell pepper, finely chopped**

¼ cup (60 ml) **white onion, finely chopped**

¼ cup (60 ml) **celery, finely chopped**

1 cup (250 ml) **portobello mushrooms, chopped**

2 tbsp **extra-virgin olive oil**

4 large **free-range eggs**

Sea salt and freshly ground pepper, to taste

1 large **tomato, cut in wedges**

5–6 spears **asparagus, trimmed**

¼ cup (60 ml) **green onion, finely chopped**

Preheat the oven to 375°F (190°C). Grease an ovenproof skillet and set aside.

In a pan, heat oil over medium heat and sauté the bell peppers, white onion, celery, and mushroom until soft and tender. Remove from heat and let cool briefly.

In a bowl, beat eggs, season with salt and pepper, add sautéed vegetables and mix well. Pour egg mixture into the greased ovenproof skillet and arrange tomato and asparagus on top. Bake in the oven for 10 minutes or until the top puffs up and is slightly golden brown.

Place fritatta onto plates, sprinkle with green onion and serve.

Serves 2

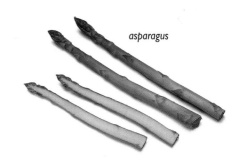

asparagus

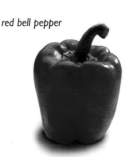

red bell pepper

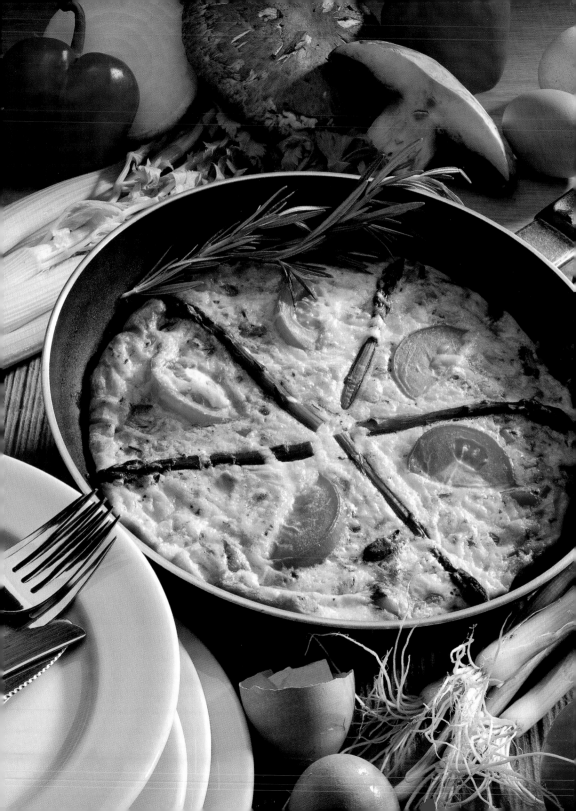

Watercress-Radish Salad

Watercress has a healing effect on the pancreas and provides abundant vitamin A, which is important to prevent the eye problems associated with diabetes.

2 cups (500 ml) **watercress**

1 cup (250 ml) **daikon radish, sliced**

½ cup (125 ml) **red radish, sliced**

1 shallot, minced

2 tbsp green onion, chopped

Dressing:

2 tbsp extra-virgin olive oil

2 tbsp cold-pressed pumpkin seed oil

3 tbsp freshly squeezed lemon juice

Sea salt and freshly ground pepper, to taste

In a large bowl, whisk together all dressing ingredients. Add all vegetables, toss well and serve.

Serves 2

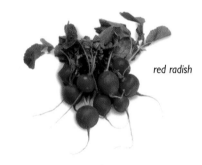

red radish

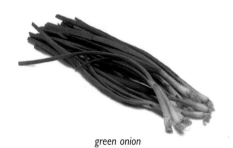

green onion

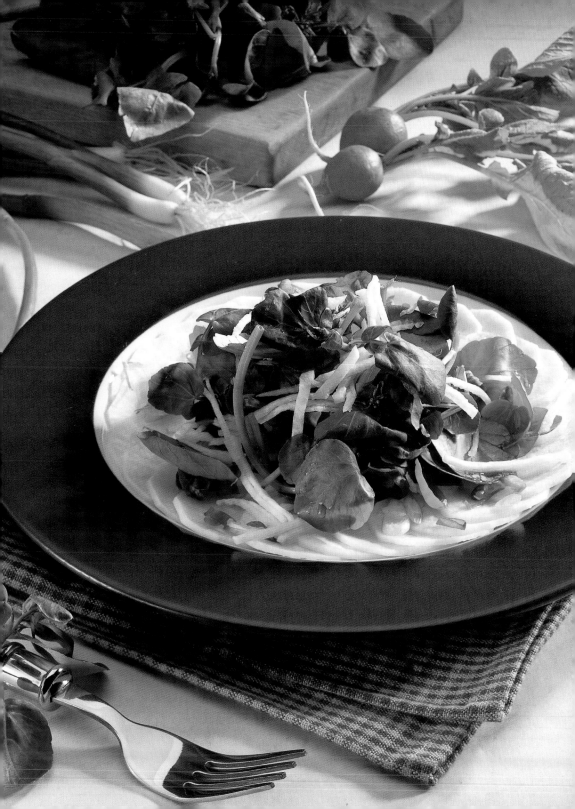

Chef's Salad with
Cream Cheese-Herb Dressing

Eaten raw, daikon, a cousin to the red radish, stimulates the gall bladder, is a diuretic, and is wonderful for digestion—all beneficial properties for treating diabetes.

2 cups (500 ml) **mixed greens**

3 **celery stalks, cut ½" (1 cm)**

1 **daikon, shredded**

1 **carrot, shredded**

1 **beefsteak tomato, cut in wedges**

½ **onion, cut in rings**

½ **English cucumber, sliced**

1 cup (250 ml) **radish, shredded**

1 cup (250 ml) **broccoli florets**

1 cup (250 ml) **cauliflower florets**

2 **soft-boiled eggs, sliced**

In a bowl, whisk together all dressing ingredients. In a separate bowl, mix together vegetables and eggs or arrange them on a platter. Pour dressing over top and serve.

Serves 2

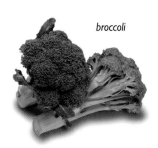

broccoli

Dressing:

¼ **cup** (60 ml) **cream cheese**

¼ **cup** (60 ml) **filtered water**

1 **tbsp freshly squeezed lemon juice**

2 **tbsp fresh herbs** (such as basil, mint, oregano)**, sliced**

2 **tbsp onion, minced**

Sea salt and freshly ground pepper, to taste

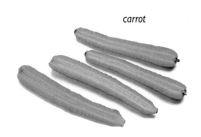

carrot

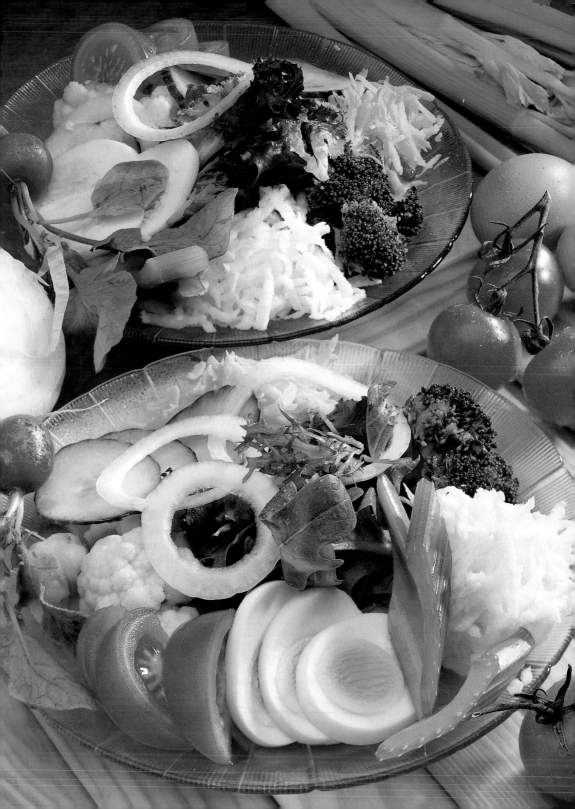

Classic Coleslaw

This simple coleslaw is easy to make and it keeps well for two or three days in the refrigerator. Keep some on hand to round out a quick and nutritious meal. Adding freshly grated apple provides crunch, flavor, and fiber in the form of pectin, which helps reverse a high blood-sugar level.

2 cups (500 ml) **white cabbage, shredded**

2 cups (500 ml) **carrots, shredded**

1 cup (250 ml) **mayonnaise**

1 organic apple, freshly grated (or pear)

1 tsp + 2 tsp freshly squeezed lemon juice

Sea salt and freshly ground pepper, to taste

Pumpkin seeds, walnuts or raisins, for garnish

In a bowl, toss the freshly grated apple in 1 teaspoon of lemon juice. In a separate large bowl, combine mayonnaise and 2 teaspoons of lemon juice. Add apple, cabbage, carrots and season with salt and pepper; mix thoroughly. Sprinkle with pumpkin seeds, walnuts or raisins, and serve.

Serves 2

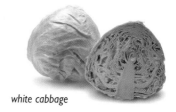

white cabbage

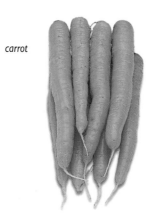

carrot

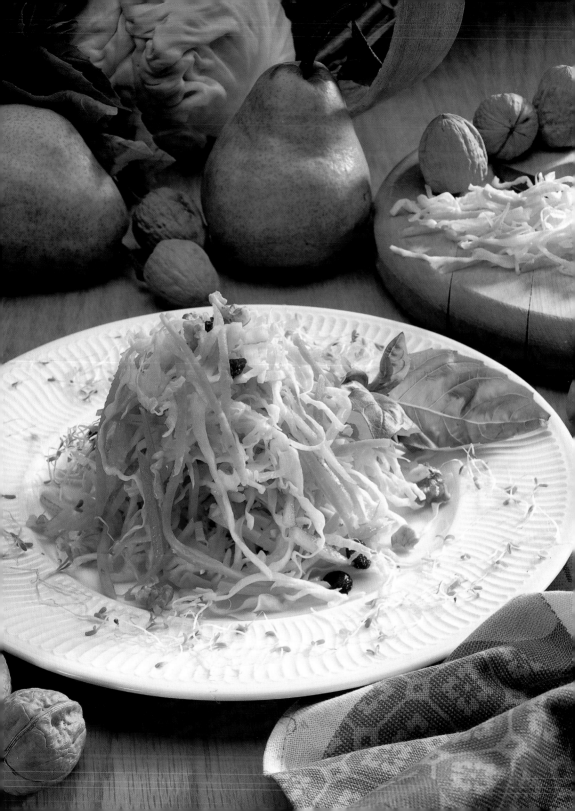

Grilled Vegetable Tower
with Watercress

The piquant flavors of the cleansing watercress and balsamic vinegar complete a colorful, eye-appealing display of wholesome vegetables.

1 tbsp + ¼ cup (60 ml) **extra-virgin olive oil**

1 large eggplant, cut in ½" (1 cm) **rounds**

1 large Bermuda onion, cut in ¼" (5 mm) **rounds**

1 large tomato, cut in ½" (1 cm) **rounds**

2 large portobello mushrooms

1 red bell pepper, quartered

Sea salt and freshly ground pepper, to taste

1 bunch watercress

1 tbsp balsamic vinegar

Carefully wipe the mushrooms clean, remove the stems and cut the tops in a checkered pattern (but not all the way through) so that the mushrooms will lie flat.

In a large pan, heat 1 tablespoon of oil over medium heat and grill each side of the eggplant, onion, tomato, mushroom, and pepper for 2 to 3 minutes or until golden brown.

Layer the grilled vegetables into towers onto plates and arrange watercress around. Drizzle remaining olive oil and balsamic vinegar over top and serve.

Serves 2

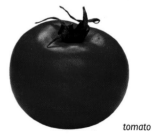

tomato

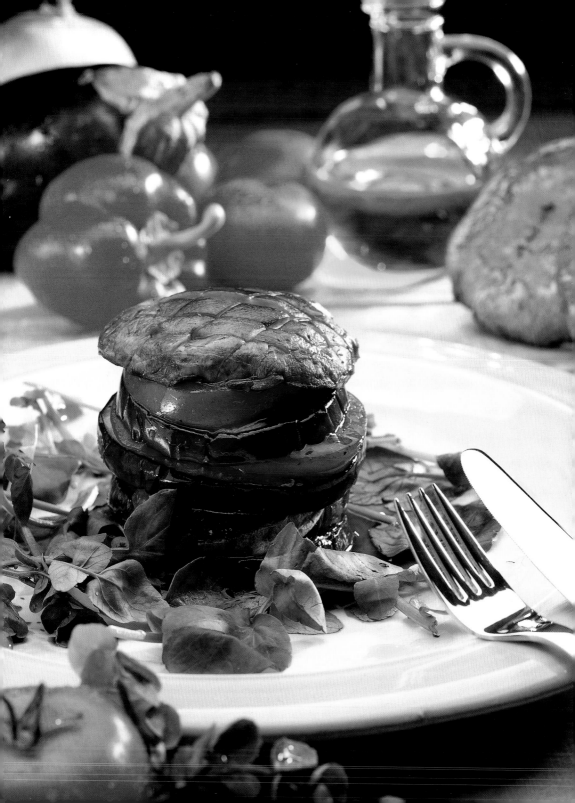

Pan-Roasted Vegetables with Poached Eggs

A diet high in vegetables will give you the fiber necessary to help contol your blood-sugar level.

1 cup (250 ml) **red onion, cut ½"** (1 cm)

2 cloves garlic, minced

2 tbsp extra-virgin olive oil

2 large carrots, cut ½" (1 cm)

1 large zucchini, cut ½" (1 cm)

1 large red bell pepper, cut ½" (1 cm)

2 celery stalks, cut ½" (1 cm)

1 cup (250 ml) **broccoli florets**

1 cup (250 ml) **cauliflower florets**

1 tbsp fresh rosemary, chopped

1 tbsp fresh sage, chopped

2 free-range eggs

1 tbsp white wine vinegar

Sea salt and freshly ground pepper, to taste

In a large pan, heat oil over medium heat and sauté onion and garlic until tender. Add remaining vegetables and sauté for 5 to 7 minutes or until tender. Stir in fresh rosemary and sage, season with salt and pepper.

In the meantime, bring a pot of water and 1 tablespoon of vinegar to a boil (the vinegar prevents the egg from separating).

Crack the eggs into the boiling water and cook for 5 to 7 minutes. Remove the eggs with a slotted spoon and drain well. Place over the vegetables and serve.

Serves 2

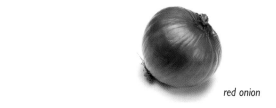

red onion

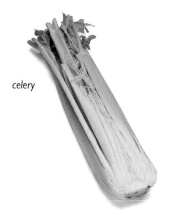

celery

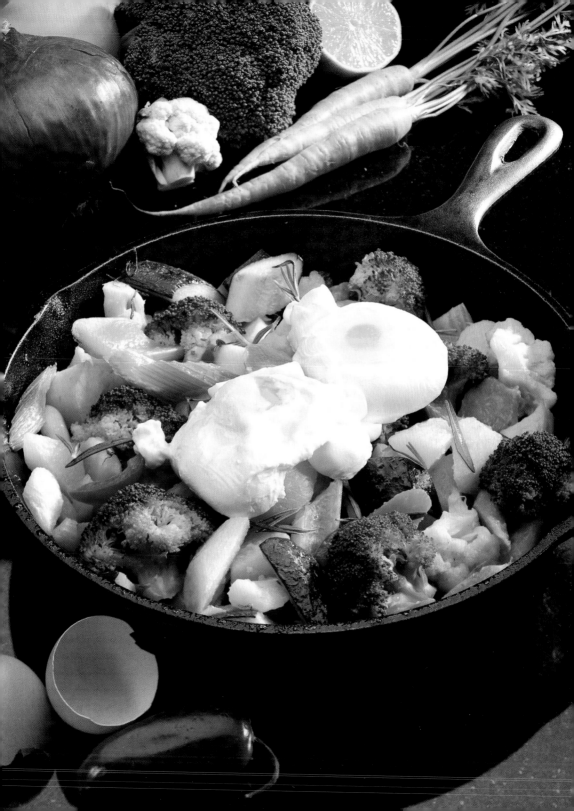

Teriyaki Tuna with Roast Potatoes

Your whole family, including children, will forget all about French fries if you offer these roast potatoes as an alternative. The teriyaki is also great with other firm ocean fish such as halibut, mahi-mahi, swordfish, or shark.

Tuna:

2 tbsp freshly squeezed lemon juice (or 1 tbsp lemon juice and 1 tbsp rice vinegar)

2 tbsp sake, rice wine or dry sherry

⅓ cup (80 ml) **soy sauce**

2 tsp fresh ginger, minced

2 cloves garlic, minced

3–4 tbsp green onion, chopped

Freshly ground black pepper, to taste

1 lb (500 g) **fresh tuna steaks**

Potatoes:

3–4 large white or russet potatoes

1–3 tsp coconut oil

½ tsp sea salt

1 tbsp cider or malt vinegar (optional)

Garlic powder, paprika, curry powder, rosemary or hot pepper powder, to taste (optional)

To prepare the tuna, combine all marinade ingredients (the first 7 ingredients) in a large bowl. Taste and adjust flavors.

Rinse fish briefly in cold water and pat dry, then place fish in a flat glass or ceramic pan. Pour marinade ingredients over fish, turning fish several times to coat. Marinate for 45 minutes at room temperature or 2 hours in refrigerator, basting and turning occasionally.

Preheat oven to 400°F (200°C). To prepare the potatoes, wash and dry them, but do not peel. Slice lengthwise like French fries or crosswise into ¼" to ½" (5 mm to 1 cm) thick slices. In a bowl, toss potato with oil, season with sea salt, and add vinegar and spices; stir gently to coat evenly.

Spread a single layer on a baking sheet and bake for 20 to 25 minutes, turning once, until golden brown and crispy (if desired). Don't worry if they stick and break up a bit, just scrape them up.

In the meantime, grill fish over medium heat on each side for 5 to 8 minutes, or until center of fish is just opaque. Serve immediately. Any leftover fish can be refrigerated, and then flaked or sliced for a delicious tuna salad the next day.

Serve tuna steaks with roast potatoes and grilled vegetables of your choice.

Serves 2

It is better to undercook fish than to overcook it. Fish does not need to flake easily to be done; it continues to cook off the grill.

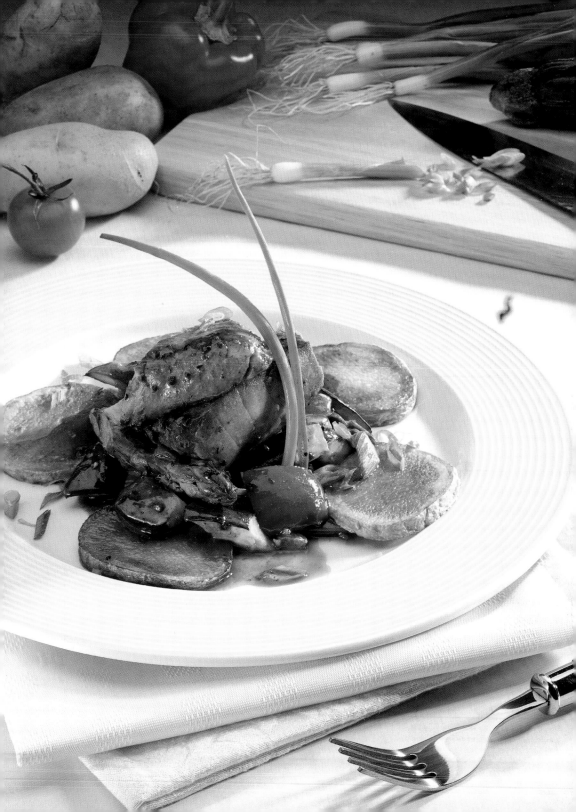

references

Anderson, J.W. et al. "Antioxidant supplementation effects on low-density lipoprotein oxidation for individuals with type 2 diabetes mellitus." *Journal of the American College of Nutrition* 18 (1999): 451-461.

Anderson, J.W. et al. "Effects of psyllium on glucose and serum lipid responses in men with type 2 diabetes and hypercholesterolemia." *American Journal of Clinical Nutrition* 70 (1999): 466-473.

Anderson, R.A. "Nutritional factors influencing the glucose/insulin system: chromium." *Journal of the American College of Nutrition* 16 (1997): 404-410.

Anderson, R.A. et al. "Elevated intakes of supplemental chromium improve glucose and insulin variables in individuals with Type 2 diabetes. *Diabetes* 46 (1997): 1786-1791.

Ashour, M. et al. "Antioxidant status and insulin-dependent diabetes mellitus (IDDM)." *Journal of Clinical Biochemistry and Nutrition* 26 (1999): 99-107.

Badmaev, V. et al. "Vanadium: A review of its potential role in the fight against diabetes." *Journal of Alternative and Complementary Medicine* 5 (1999): 273-291.

Baynes, J.W. and Thorpe, S.R. "Role of oxidative stress in diabetic complications: a new prospective on an old paradigm." *Diabetes* 48 (1999): 1-9.

Boden, G. et al. "Effects of vanadyl sulfate on carbohydrate and lipid metabolism in patients with non-insulin-dependent diabetes mellitus." *Metabolism* 45 (1996): 1130-1135.

Bursell, S.E. et al. "High-dose vitamin E supplementation normalizes retinal blood flow and creatinine clearance in patients with Type I diabetes." *Diabetes Care* 22 (1998): 1245-1251.

Carter, J.S. et al. "Non-insulin dependent diabetes mellitus in minorities in the United States." *Annals of Internal Medicine* 125 (1996): 221-232.

Cefalu, W.T. et al. "Effect of chromium picolinate on insulin sensitivity in vivo". *Journal of Trace Elements in Experimental Medicine* 12 (1999): 71-83.

Ceriello, A. et al. "Antioxidant defences are reduced during the orla glucose tolerance test in normal and non-insulin-dependent diabetic subjects." *European Journal of Clinical Investigation* 28 (1998): 329-333.

Connor, W.E. "_-linolenic acid in health and disease." *American Journal of Clinical Nutrition* 69 (1999): 827-828.

Crook, W.G. *The Yeast Connection and the Woman.* Jackson, TN: Professional Books, 1999.

Cunnane, S.C. et al. "High _-linoleic flaxseed (linum usitaissimum): some nutritional properties." *British Journal of Nutrition* 69 (1993): 443-453.

Cunningham, J.J. "The glucose/insulin system and vitamin C: implications in insulin-dependent diabetes mellitus." *Journal of the American College of Nutrition* 17 (1998): 105-108.

Ding, W. et al. "Serum and urine chromium concentrations in elderly diabetics." *Biological Trace Element Research* 63 (1998): 231-237.

Editors. "Effects of a short-term circuit weight training program on glycemic control in NIDDM." *Diabetes Research and Clinical Practice* 40: 53-61.

Eriksson J. and Kohvakka, A. "Magnesium and ascorbic acid supplementation in diabetes mellitus." *Annals of Nutrition and Metabolism* 39 (1995): 217-223.

Eriksson, J.G. "Exercise and the treatment of Type 2 diabetes mellitus: an update." *Sports Medicine* 27 (1995): 381-391.

Garlic, A. et al. "Intracellular magnesium depletion relates to increased urinary magnesium loss in Type I diabetes." *Hormone and Metabolic Research* 30 (1998): 99-102.

Geliebter et al. "Effects of strength or aerobic training on body composition, resting metabolic rate, and peak oxygen consumption in obese dieting subjects." *American Journal of Clinical Nutrition* 66 (1998): 557-563.

Gerster, H. "Can adults adequately convert _-linolenic acid (18:3n-3) to eicosapetaenaoic acid (20:5n-3) and docosahexaenoic acid (22:6n-3)?" *International Journal of Vitamin and Trace Element Research* 68 (1998): 159-173.

Hancke, J.L. et al. "Schizandra chinensis (Turcz.) Baill." *Fitoterapia* 70 (1997): 451-471.

Head, K.A. "Type-I diabetes: prevention of the disease and its complications." *Alternative Medicine Review* 2 (1997): 256-281.

Horrobin, D.F. "Essential fatty acids in the management of impaired nerve function in diabetes." *Diabetes* 46 (Suppl. 2) (1997): S90-S93.

Ivy, J.L. "Role of exercise training in the prevention and treatment of insulin resistance and non-insulin-dependent-diabetes mellitus." *Sports Medicine* 24 (1997): 321-336.

Jain, S.K. et al. "Relationship of blood thromboxane-B2 (TXB2) with lipid peroxides and effect of vitamin E and placebo supplementation on TXB2 and lipid peroxide levels in Type I diabetic patients." *Diabetes Care* 21 (1998): 1511-1516.

Li, Al et al. "Hemorheology and walking of peripheral arterial occlusive diseases patients during treatment with *Ginkgo biloba* extract." *Chung Kuo Yao Li Hsueh Pao* 19 (1998): 417-421.

Macor, C. et al. "Visceral adipose tissue impairs insulin secretion and insulin sensitivity but not energy expenditure in obesity." *Metabolism* 46 (1997): 123-129.

McAuliffe, A.V. et al. "Administration of ascorbic acid and an aldose reductase inhibitor (Tolrestat) in diabetes: effect on urinary albumin excretion." *Nephron* 80 (1998): 277-284.

McKeigue, P.M. et al. "Relation of central obesity and insulin resistance with high diabetes prevalence and cardiovascular risk in South Asians." *Lancet* 337 (1991): 382-386.

Miller, A.L. and Kelly, G.S. "Homocysteine metabolism: nutritional modulation and impact on health and disease." *Alternative Medicine Review* 2 (1997): 234-254.

Pan, D.A. et al. "Skeletal muscle membrane lipid composition is related to adiposity and insulin action." *Journal of Clinical Investigation* 96 (1995): 2802-2808.

Paolisso, G. et al. "Pharmacological doses of vitamin E improve insulin action in healthy subjects and non-insulin-dependent diabetic patients." *American Journal of Clinical Nutrition* 57 (1993): 650-656.

Raman, A. and Lau, A. "Anti-diabetic properties and phytochemistry of Momordica chantaria L. (Curcubitacea)." *Phytomedicine* 2 (1996): 349-362.

Ravina, A. et al. "Reversal of corticosteroid-induced diabetes mellitus with supplemental chromium." *Diabetic Medicine* 16 (1999): 164-167.

Rodriguez-Moran, M. et al. "Lipid and glucose-lowering efficacy of Plantago psyllium in type II diabetes." *Journal of Diabetes Complications* 12 (1998): 273-278.

Rogers, K.S. and Mohan, C. "Vitamin B6 metabolism and diabetes." *Biochemical Medicine and Metabolic Biology* 52 (1994): 10-17.

Sajithlal, G.B. et al. "Effect of curcumin on the advanced glycation and cross linking of collagen in diabetic rats." *Biochemical Pharmacology* 56 (1998): 1607-1614.

Salmeron, J. et al. "Dietary fiber, glycemic load, and risk of non-insulin dependent diabetes mellitus in women." *Journal of the American Medical Association* 77 (1997): 472-477.

references

Serraclara, A. et al. "Hypoglycemic action of an oral fig-leaf decoction in type-I diabetic patients." *Diabetes Research and Clinical Practice* 39, (1998): 19-22.

Sharma, R.D. et al. "Hypolipidaemic effect of fenugreek seeds: a chronic study in non-insulin dependent diabetic patients." *Phytotherapy Research* 10 (1996): 332-334.

Sirtori, C. et al. "n-3 fatty acids do not lead to an increased diabetic risk in patients with hyperlipidemia and abnormal glucose tolerance." *American Journal of Clinical Nutrition* 65 (1997): 1874-1881.

Soto, P. et al. "Prevention of alloxan-induced diabetes mellitus in the rat by silymarin." *Comparative Biochemistry and Physiology C: Pharmacology, Toxicology and Endocrinology* 119 (1998): 126-129.

Srimal, R.C. "Turmeric: A brief review of medicinal properties." *Fitoterapia* 6 (1997): 483-493.

Storlien, L.H. et al. "Influence of dietary fat composition on development of insulin resistance in rats." *Diabetes* 40 (1991): 280-289.

Tessier, D. et al. "Effects of an oral glucose challenge on free radicals/antioxidants balance in an older population with Type II diabetes." *Journal of Gerontology A: Biological Science and Medical Science* 54 (1999): M541-M545.

Timimi, F.K. et al. "Vitamin C improved endothelium-dependent vasodilationin patients with insulin-dependent diabetes mellitus." *Journal of the American College of Cardiology* 31 (1998): 552-557.

Tutuncu, N.B. et al. "The effect of vitamin E supplementation on erthyrocyte osmotic fragility in diabetic patients." *Clinical Hemorheology and Microcirculation* 20 (1999): 201-207.

Vaarala, O. et al. "Environmental factors in the aetiology of childhood diabetes." Diabetes, Nutrition and Metabolism (1999).

Velussi, et al. Long-term (12 months) treatment with an anti-oxidant drug (silymarin) is effective on hyperinsulinemia, exogenous insulin need and malondialdehyde levels in cirrhotic diabetic patients." *Journal of Hepatology* 26 (1997): 871-879.

Will, J.C. et al. "Serum vitamin C concentrations and diabetes: Findings from the Third National Health and Nutrition Examination Survey, 1988-1994." *American Journal of Clinical Nutrition* 70 (1999): 49-52.

Zeigler, D. and Gries, F.A. "_-lipoic acid in the treatment of diabetic peripheral and autonomic neuropathy." *Diabetes* 46 (Suppl. 2) (1997): S62-S66.

Zhang, J.Q. et al. "Effects of silybin on red blood cell sorbitol and nerve conduction velocity in diabetic patients." *Chung Kuo Chung His I Chieh Ho Tsa Chih* 13 (1993): 708, 725-726.

sources

Flora
7400 Fraser Park Drive
Burnaby BC V5J 5B9
(604) 436–6000
1-800-663-0617 (Western Canada)
1-800-387-7541 (Eastern Canada)

Hempola
3405 American Dr. #5
Mississauga, Ontario, Canada
L4V 1T6
Tel: 1-800-240-9215
Tel: (905) 678-1066
Fax: (905) 678-6036
Website: www.hempola.com

Nature's Life
7180 Lampson Ave
Garden Grove CA 92841-3914
(714) 379–6500
1-800-854-6837 or 1-800-338-7979
www.nutritionexpress.com

Omega Nutrition of Canada, Inc.
1924 Franklin Street
Vancouver BC V5L 1R2
(604) 253–4677
1-800-661-3529
www.omegaflo.com

Stoney Creek Oil Products Pty. Ltd.
Talbot, Victoria, Australia 3371
Tel: (03) 5463 2340

First published in 2000 by
alive **books**
7436 Fraser Park Drive
Burnaby BC V5J 5B9
(604) 435–1919
1-800–661–0303

© 2000 by *alive* books

Book Design:
 Liza Novecoski
Artwork:
 Terence Yeung
 Raymond Cheung
Food Styling/Recipe Development:
 Fred Edrissi
Photography:
 Edmond Fong (recipe photos)
 Siegfried Gursche
Photo Editing:
 Sabine Edrissi-Bredenbrock
Editing:
 Sandra Tonn

Canadian Cataloguing in Publication Data

Broadhurst, C. Leigh
 Prevent, Treat and
 Reverse Diabetes

(*alive* natural health guides, 24
ISSN 1490-6503)
ISBN 1-55312-020-5

Printed in Canada

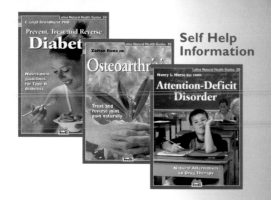
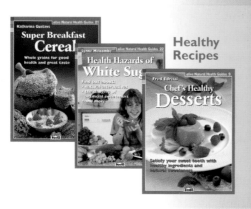
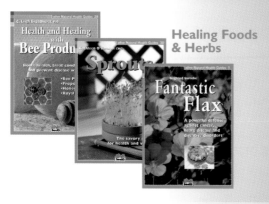
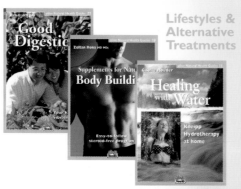